Post Traumatic Growth

Rebuilding the Nervous System, Identity, and Meaning After Trauma

By Jim Moltzan

Disclaimer

This book is intended for informational and educational purposes only. It is not a substitute for professional medical, psychological, or mental health treatment. Nothing in this book should be interpreted as medical advice, mental health diagnosis, clinical intervention, or a guarantee of outcome. Readers experiencing significant emotional distress, trauma symptoms, or health concerns should consult a qualified healthcare or mental health professional.

The practices and concepts presented herein are offered as general guidance. The author does not promise or imply any specific results, nor is the author responsible for any adverse outcomes arising from the use or misuse of the information contained in this book. Use the material at your own discretion and risk.

The author has made every effort to ensure accuracy and completeness. However, the author makes no representations or warranties regarding the applicability, fitness, or completeness of the content for any individual reader.

This book is © copyrighted by CAD Graphics, Inc. No part of this publication may be copied, altered, sold, or used in any form beyond what is permitted by law. No portion may be reproduced or transmitted in any form or by any means whether graphic, electronic, or mechanical, including photocopying, recording, or any information storage and retrieval system, without the written permission of the author.

© 2025 CAD Graphics, Inc.

ISBN: 978-1-958837-52-8

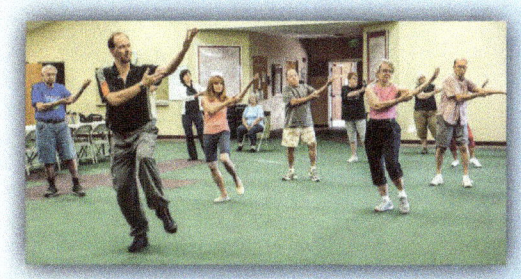 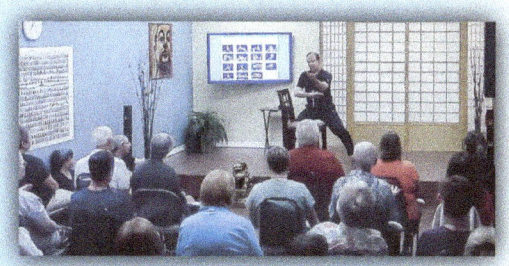
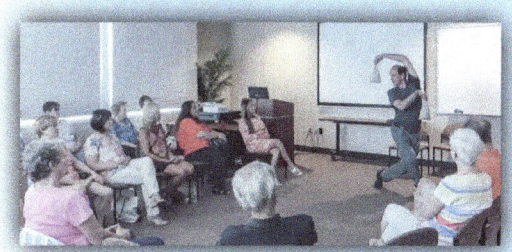 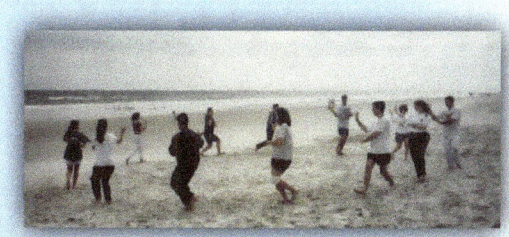
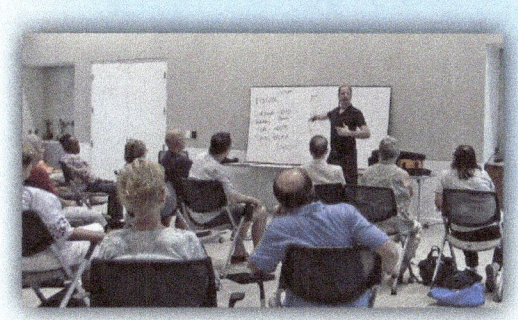 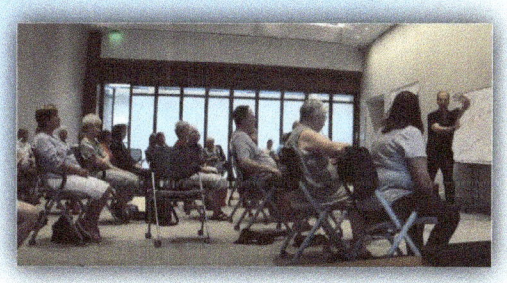
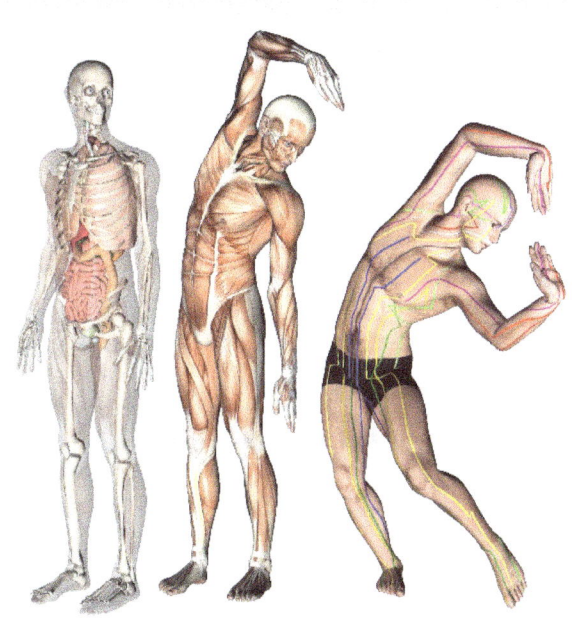

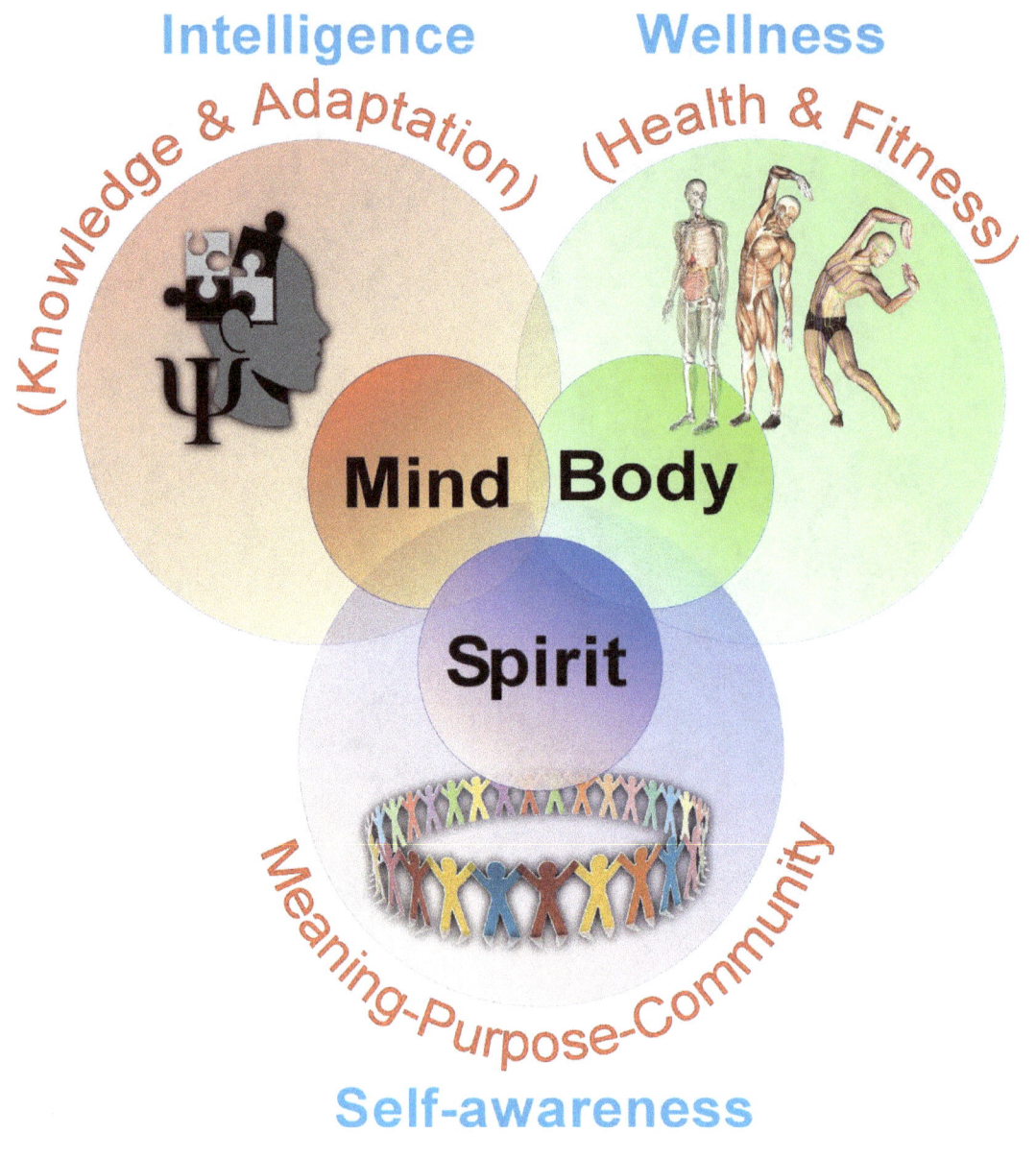

We are the architect of our own health, happiness, destiny, or fate.

Table of Contents

Preface 1
Acknowledgments 2
Author's Note 3

Part I — Foundations of Trauma and Growth 4
   Chapter 1 - Trauma, Conditioning, and the Search for Wholeness 5
   Chapter 2 - "The Somatic Foundation of Recovery 9
   Chapter 3 - Cognitive Recovery 15
   Chapter 4 - Emotional Integration 21

Part II — The Physiology of Healing and Self-Regulation 28
   Chapter 5 - Breath, Posture, and Nervous System Regulation in Post-Traumatic Growth 29
   Chapter 6 - Practical Methods of Emotional and Physiological Self-Regulation 42
   Chapter 7 - Rewiring the Stress Response 49

Part III — Identity, Meaning, and Psychological Integration 81
   Chapter 8 - Boundaries, Discernment, and Psychological Autonomy 82
   Chapter 9 - Meaning-Making, Purpose, and Identity Reconstruction After Trauma ... 89
   Chapter 10 - Shadow Work, Emotional Maturity, and Post-Traumatic Growth 96
   Chapter 11 - Conflict, Attachment Triggers, and Relational Healing 103

Part IV — Growth, Contribution, and Life Reintegration 110
   Chapter 12 - Expanded Self-Awareness and Psychological Maturity 111
   Chapter 13 - Reclaiming Agency, Choice, and Life Direction 118
   Chapter 14 - Service, Contribution, and the Mature Expression of Growth 125
   Chapter 15 - Integration, Wholeness, and the Ongoing Growth Process 132

Part VII – Appendices & Resources 139
   Appendix A – Nervous Systems 140
   Appendix B - Box Breathing: A Method to Manage Stress 142
   Appendix C – Other Breathing Patterns 145
   Appendix D - Qigong 148
   Appendix E – 5 Element Qigong 152
   Appendix F – Concept of Kan and Li 154
   Appendix G – Small Circulation Exercises 156
   Appendix H – 8 Pieces of Brocade 160

Appendix I – Chamsa Meditation 164

Appendix J – A Metaphorical Lens on Interpersonal Stress and Support 170

Glossary 176

Glossary - Graphic 182

About the Instructor, Author & Artist - Jim Moltzan 186

Books Available Through Amazon 188

Contacts 190

Preface

Trauma rarely arrives by invitation. For most people, it enters life unexpectedly, through loss, betrayal, illness, accidents, violence, neglect, coercion, or prolonged stress. Very few individuals seek out traumatic experiences, and just as rarely do most people consciously intend to harm or traumatize others. And yet, despite intent, all actions carry consequences. Words spoken in anger, choices made in fear, systems built on imbalance, and moments of inattention can send ripple effects outward for years, sometimes for generations. Trauma often lives in these ripples.

Long after the original event has passed, many people continue to feel unsettled inside, anxious, guarded, emotionally numb, reactive, ashamed, or unsure of who they have become. These experiences are not signs of weakness or personal failure. They are the natural imprint of overwhelming stress on the nervous system, identity, and relational trust. Trauma changes how the body responds to threat, how the mind interprets reality, how the self is organized, and how relationships are navigated.

This book was written for those who have survived difficult experiences and now find themselves asking deeper questions, not only *how to cope*, but how to truly **grow beyond survival**. Post-traumatic growth does not mean that trauma was good, necessary, deserved, or spiritually justified. It does not minimize suffering or attempt to frame pain as a gift. Rather, it acknowledges a well-documented truth: human beings possess a powerful capacity to adapt, integrate, mature, and rebuild their lives when safety, awareness, and agency are gradually restored.

For decades, my work has focused on the relationship between **stress physiology, emotional regulation, behavior, identity, and resilience**. Again and again, I have seen that trauma recovery is not only psychological. It is neurological. It is relational. It is embodied. Insight alone is not enough. Healing requires the reorganization of the nervous system, the development of emotional maturity, the rebuilding of boundaries, the restoration of agency, and the reconstruction of meaning.

This book follows the full arc of transformation. It begins with how trauma disrupts regulation, perception, and identity. It then moves into the practical foundations of recovery—breath, posture, emotional regulation, and stress resilience. From there, it addresses the deeper psychological work of boundaries, meaning-making, emotional maturity, and agency. Finally, it turns outward toward contribution, service, and the lifelong process of integration and wholeness.

If you are reading this, it is likely because some part of your life has been shaped by adversity, sudden or prolonged, visible or hidden. This book does not offer shortcuts. It offers something more enduring: a grounded path toward rebuilding stability, identity, agency, and meaning over time.

Growth does not erase the past. It allows you to live no longer defined by it.

Acknowledgments

This book reflects not only years of study, practice, and writing, but the influence of many people who, in different ways, shaped the path that led to these pages. While this work focuses on trauma, growth, and recovery, it also stands as a quiet acknowledgment of the relationships, teachers, students, and lived experiences that made such an exploration possible.

I am deeply grateful to those who have shared their stories with me over the years, often at great personal cost and with remarkable courage. Your willingness to speak openly about suffering, resilience, confusion, and transformation has continually deepened my understanding of what post-traumatic growth truly looks like in lived experience. This book is, in many ways, a reflection of that collective wisdom.

I also acknowledge the many teachers, mentors, and researchers, both within and beyond the fields of psychology, neuroscience, and human development, whose work has provided a scientific and ethical foundation for this manuscript. The body of trauma-informed research now available has transformed how we understand the nervous system, identity, attachment, and recovery. I am grateful for those who pursued this work with rigor, humility, and compassion.

To my students and clients, past and present: thank you for the trust you placed in me during some of the most challenging periods of your lives. You taught me that healing is not linear, that strength often appears quietly, and that transformation rarely looks the way we expect it to. Your perseverance continues to inform my work more than any single theory or method.

I am also grateful for the support of friends and colleagues who encourage my many writing projects during their many stages of development. Writing about trauma and growth is demanding work, and your steady presence, honest feedback, and patience mattered more than you know.

Finally, I acknowledge the quiet inner work that accompanies any long creative and reflective process, in the revisions, false starts, and perseverance that no reader ever sees. This book exists because of that sustained effort and the conviction that understanding leads to freedom.

If these pages offer clarity, steadiness, or hope to even one person navigating their own recovery, then every step of the journey that brought this book into being has been worth it.

Author's Note

My work has been shaped by more than four decades of study, practice, and teaching in the fields of martial arts, internal movement systems, breath training, stress physiology, and holistic human development. I began training in the traditional martial arts at a young age, and over time my path expanded to include Tai Chi, Qigong, Dao Yin, stance training, conditioning methods, and meditative movement practices. These systems taught me through direct experience what modern neuroscience now confirms: the body is not separate from the mind. Posture, breath, movement, and attention are inseparable from emotional regulation, perception, and behavior.

Alongside physical training, I pursued formal academic study in holistic health, psychology, human behavior, and integrative wellness. Over the years, this dual path, embodied training and clinical understanding, led me to a central realization: trauma is not simply an emotional or psychological event. It is a **whole-system experience** that reshapes the nervous system, alters identity, reorganizes relationships, and influences meaning itself. This understanding has guided both my teaching and my writing, and it forms the foundation of the framework presented in this book.

Throughout my career, I have worked with individuals from many backgrounds, such as athletes, military veterans, survivors of abuse, those living under chronic stress, and people simply seeking greater clarity and stability in their lives. Again and again, I have witnessed how regulation of breath, restoration of posture, and disciplined movement open the doorway to emotional steadiness, psychological maturity, and personal agency. These are not theories to me. They are patterns I have observed unfold across thousands of hours of instruction, practice, failure, recovery, and human encounter.

In my broader body of work, I have articulated what I call the **Warrior, Scholar, and Sage** archetype system. These three roles represent the integrated cultivation of physical discipline (Warrior), intellectual discernment (Scholar), and ethical wisdom (Sage). While this book does not focus on that framework directly, its influence is quietly present throughout. Post-traumatic growth ultimately asks the same timeless questions these archetypes have always addressed: *How do we train ourselves when life has wounded us? How do we understand ourselves when identity has been shaken? And how do we live with integrity after suffering has altered our path?*

This book is not offered as a doctrine or an answer to every question. It is offered as a companion for those navigating the demanding, deeply human work of rebuilding stability, meaning, and wholeness after trauma.

- Jim Moltzan

Part I — Foundations of Trauma and Growth

Chapter 1 - Trauma, Conditioning, and the Search for Wholeness

Trauma is not defined solely by catastrophic events. It is defined by how the nervous system responds to overwhelming experiences that exceed a person's capacity to cope at the time they occur. Trauma can emerge from abuse, neglect, betrayal, humiliation, coercion, abandonment, chronic stress, accidents, medical crises, high-control environments, warfare, or long-term emotional suppression. What unites these experiences is not the event itself, but the persistent imprint they leave on perception, memory, emotion, identity, and physiological regulation (Herman, 1992; van der Kolk, 2014).

Trauma reshapes how people interpret safety, danger, trust, power, and self-worth. It fragments the continuity of experience and disrupts the internal story a person tells about who they are and how the world works. Survivors often emerge from trauma with heightened vigilance, emotional volatility, dissociation, chronic anxiety, depression, or persistent feelings of shame and disorientation (American Psychiatric Association, 2022). These patterns are not signs of weakness. They are adaptive survival responses encoded in the nervous system.

Yet trauma does not only disrupt. Under the right conditions, it can also become the catalyst for profound psychological growth. This process is known as **post-traumatic growth (PTG)**, a term that describes the development of greater personal strength, emotional depth, relational capacity, meaning, and purpose following adversity (Tedeschi & Calhoun, 2004, 2018). Growth does not occur because trauma is good. Growth occurs because the human nervous system and psyche possess an inherent drive toward coherence when safety, awareness, and support are restored.

The central question of recovery is not simply, "How do I eliminate symptoms?" It is, "How do I become whole again?" Healing is not a return to the person one used to be. It is the construction of a new self, informed by experience, strengthened by insight, and guided by clarity rather than fear (McAdams, 2013; Park, 2010).

Trauma as Nervous System Imprinting

When overwhelming stress occurs, the brain prioritizes survival over reflection. The amygdala activates threat detection, the autonomic nervous system shifts into fight, flight, or shutdown, and higher reasoning becomes secondary. In these moments, memory is stored not as a coherent narrative but as fragmented sensory impressions, bodily tension patterns, emotional surges, and implicit beliefs about safety and danger (LeDoux, 2012; van der Kolk, 2014).

Long after the original threat has passed, the nervous system may continue to behave as if danger remains present. This results in hypervigilance, exaggerated startle responses, emotional flooding, numbness, intrusive memories, chronic pain, sleep disturbances, or persistent fatigue (Herman, 1992; Porges, 2011). These are not psychological flaws. They are remnants of a nervous system that learned to survive under pressure.

Trauma also conditions perception. Survivors may begin to see threats where none exists, minimize their own needs, struggle with boundaries, tolerate harmful environments, or unconsciously repeat relational dynamics that mirror earlier wounds. These patterns are not chosen. They are learned through repeated activation of survival circuitry (Siegel, 2012; van der Kolk, 2014).

Conditioning and the Loss of Psychological Sovereignty

In many cases, trauma is compounded by **conditioning,** or the gradual shaping of belief systems, self-concept, and behavior through repetition, authority, fear, reward, and social pressure. Conditioning can occur in families, institutions, religious systems, cultic environments, abusive relationships, workplaces, and even algorithm-driven digital platforms (Haidt, 2024; Lifton, 1989).

When conditioning is based on coercion rather than autonomy, individuals may lose psychological sovereignty. They may internalize external voices, adopt beliefs that contradict their lived experience, suppress emotional truth, or doubt their own perceptions. Over time, this erodes self-trust and fragments identity (Herman, 1992; Lifton, 1989).

Recovery from trauma therefore requires more than calming symptoms. It requires the restoration of **self-authorship**, or the ability to think, feel, choose, and interpret reality from one's own grounded center (Siegel, 2012; McAdams, 2013).

The Drive Toward Wholeness

Despite the disruptions caused by trauma, the human organism retains an innate drive toward integration. This drive is expressed through the desire to make meaning, restore coherence, reconnect with others, and live with purpose. Even when survivors feel broken, exhausted, or disconnected, the impulse toward healing remains active beneath the surface (Park, 2010; Frankl, 2006).

Wholeness does not mean the absence of scars. It means that scars no longer govern perception, identity, or choice. It means that memory becomes integrated into narrative rather than trapped in the body as tension and reactivity. It means the nervous system regains flexibility instead of remaining locked in survival mode (Siegel, 2012; van der Kolk, 2014).

Post-traumatic growth occurs when survivors begin to experience:

- A deeper appreciation for life

- Increased personal strength
- More authentic relationships
- Expanded emotional awareness
- Greater clarity of values
- A revised sense of purpose
- A broader understanding of suffering and resilience

(Tedeschi & Calhoun, 2004, 2018).

Growth does not erase pain. It transforms how pain is held within the psyche.

From Survival to Growth

In early recovery, survival remains the dominant organizing principle. The nervous system scans for threat. The body holds tension. The mind anticipates danger. Over time, with the right interventions, the system begins to soften. Safety becomes internally generated rather than externally dependent. Regulation replaces reactivity. Discernment replaces fear-based interpretation (Porges, 2011; Siegel, 2012).

This transition marks the shift from **trauma adaptation** to **post-traumatic growth**. It is not a sudden leap. It is a gradual reorganization of body, mind, and identity (Tedeschi & Calhoun, 2018).

This book is designed to guide that reorganization.

The Structure of Growth in This Book

This work follows four progressive stages:

1. Understanding trauma and its effects
2. Regulating the nervous system through breath, posture, and somatic awareness
3. Reconstructing identity, meaning, and psychological boundaries
4. Integrating growth into relationships, contribution, and life direction

Each stage builds upon the previous one. None can be skipped. Growth is cumulative and layered (Herman, 1992; Siegel, 2012).

The Work Begins Here

The path forward does not demand perfection. It does not require spiritual belief, philosophical adherence, or blind optimism. It requires only willingness, self-honesty, and consistent practice. Healing is not achieved through force. It unfolds through patience, regulation, insight, and relational safety (van der Kolk, 2014; Frankl, 2006).

What was once endured as survival can become, with time and integration, the foundation for strength, depth, and mature compassion (Tedeschi & Calhoun, 2018).

REFERENCES — CHAPTER 1

American Psychiatric Association. (2022). *Diagnostic and statistical manual of mental disorders* (5th ed., text rev.; DSM-5-TR). American Psychiatric Publishing.

Frankl, V. E. (2006). *Man's search for meaning* (Rev. ed.). Beacon Press. (Original work published 1946)

Haidt, J. (2024). The anxious generation: How the great rewiring of childhood is causing an epidemic of mental illness. Penguin Press.

Herman, J. L. (1992). Trauma and recovery: The aftermath of violence—from domestic abuse to political terror. Basic Books.

LeDoux, J. (2012). *Rethinking the emotional brain*. Neuron, 73(4), 653–676. https://doi.org/10.1016/j.neuron.2012.02.004

Lifton, R. J. (1989). Thought reform and the psychology of totalism: A study of brainwashing in China. University of North Carolina Press.

McAdams, D. P. (2013). *The redemptive self: Stories Americans live by* (Revised and expanded ed.). Oxford University Press.

Park C. L. (2010). Making sense of the meaning literature: an integrative review of meaning making and its effects on adjustment to stressful life events. *Psychological bulletin*, *136*(2), 257–301. https://doi.org/10.1037/a0018301

Porges, S. W. (2011). The polyvagal theory: Neurophysiological foundations of emotions, attachment, communication, and self-regulation. W. W. Norton & Company.

Siegel, D. J. (2012). The developing mind: How relationships and the brain interact to shape who we are (2nd ed.). Guilford Press.

Tedeschi, R.G., Shakespeare-Finch, J., & Taku, K. (2018). Posttraumatic Growth: Theory, Research, and Applications (1st ed.). Routledge. https://doi.org/10.4324/9781315527451

Tedeschi, R. G., & Calhoun, L. G. (2018). Posttraumatic growth: Theory, research, and applications. Routledge.

van der Kolk, B. A. (2014). The body keeps the score: Brain, mind, and body in the healing of trauma. Viking.

Chapter 2 - "The Somatic Foundation of Recovery

Strength, Safety, and Embodied Stability

Trauma is not only a psychological experience. It is a physiological condition that reshapes how the body organizes movement, posture, breath, tension, and internal sensation. Long after the original threat has passed, the body may continue to live as if danger is still present. Muscles remain guarded, breathing becomes shallow, posture collapses or stiffens, and interoceptive awareness narrows. These bodily adaptations are not symbolic. They are survival strategies embedded in the nervous system (van der Kolk, 2014; Porges, 2011).

For this reason, recovery cannot occur solely through insight or talk-based therapy. Healing must be built on a **somatic foundation**, meaning that safety, strength, and stability must first be restored in the body. Without this foundation, higher cognitive and emotional work lacks support. The body remains reactive, even when the mind understands what has happened.

> **Post-traumatic growth begins when the body learns that the danger has passed.**

Trauma as a Disorder of Regulation

At its core, trauma is a disorder of autonomic regulation. The autonomic nervous system governs heart rate, digestion, breathing, blood pressure, immune response, and emotional reactivity. When a person is exposed to overwhelming stress, the system shifts into survival modes dominated by:

- Sympathetic activation (fight or flight)
- Dorsal vagal shutdown (collapse, numbness, dissociation)

(Porges, 2011).

In healthy functioning, the nervous system moves flexibly between states of activation and rest. Trauma disrupts this rhythm. Survivors may become trapped in chronic hyperarousal (anxiety, anger, vigilance) or chronic hypoarousal (fatigue, numbness, depression). This dysregulation affects cognition, relationships, emotional control, immune health, sleep, and pain perception (van der Kolk, 2014; Siegel, 2012). Somatic recovery is the process of restoring this lost flexibility.

Safety as a Physiological Experience

Safety is not a belief. It is a **body-based state**. A person can tell themselves they are safe, yet their heart rate, muscle tension, breathing, and visceral sensations may still signal danger. This internal mismatch creates confusion, emotional instability, and exhaustion.

Neuroscience shows that the brain evaluates safety primarily through:

- Breath rhythm
- Postural tone
- Facial expression
- Voice prosody
- Muscle tension
- Visceral sensation

(Porges, 2011; Siegel, 2012).

Until these systems stabilize, the brain cannot consistently differentiate past threat from present reality.

Therefore, establishing safety in the body is the first task of recovery.

This is accomplished through:

- Breath regulation
- Grounded posture
- Gentle strength-building
- Slow, intentional movement
- Interoceptive awareness

These are not secondary practices. They are primary biological interventions.

Posture and the Architecture of Stability

Posture is one of the most powerful and overlooked determinants of emotional regulation. A collapsed posture compresses the lungs, restricts the diaphragm, decreases oxygenation, and increases threat signaling to the brain. Conversely, upright, supported posture enhances confidence, memory, affect regulation, and resilience (Peper et al., 2016).

Trauma survivors frequently adopt defensive postures such as:

- Rounded shoulders
- Forward head position
- Contracted abdomen
- Restricted rib movement
- Locked hips or knees

These patterns reflect a nervous system organized around protection rather than engagement.

Corrective posture work improves:

- Vagal tone
- Balance
- Emotional resilience
- Pain regulation
- Cognitive clarity
- Self-efficacy

(Peper et al., 2016; Porges, 2011).

Postural restoration is therefore a direct intervention into trauma physiology.

Strength as a Regulator of the Nervous System

Strength training is not only a musculoskeletal intervention. It is a **neuroregulatory tool**. Resistance training increases:

- Neuroplasticity
- Stress tolerance
- Dopamine and serotonin regulation
- Sleep quality
- Mood stability
- Executive functioning

(Ratey & Loehr, 2011; Dishman et al., 2006).

For trauma survivors, physical strength carries additional psychological benefits:

- Restores a sense of agency
- Rebuilds trust in the body
- Increases perceived self-efficacy
- Reduces helplessness
- Enhances emotional containment

Strength training teaches the nervous system that effort can be survived, discomfort can be tolerated, and capacity can expand safely.

This process directly supports post-traumatic growth by restoring competence and confidence at the physiological level.

Grounding and Interoceptive Awareness

Grounding refers to the ability to remain connected to present-moment bodily sensation. Trauma disrupts this capacity through dissociation, numbing, or hyperreactivity.

Survivors may feel disconnected from their bodies or overwhelmed by bodily sensation. Interoception, the brain's ability to interpret internal bodily signals, is central to emotional regulation (Critchley & Harrison, 2013). When interoception is impaired:

- Emotional states become confusing
- Panic emerges without clear cause
- Fatigue becomes chronic
- Identity feels unstable

Grounding practices restore interoception through:

- Slow standing exercises
- Weight-shifting
- Conscious walking
- Gentle pressure through the feet
- Tactile awareness
- Breath-attuned movement

These methods anchor awareness in the present and reduce dissociative drift (Ogden et al., 2006; van der Kolk, 2014).

Breath as the Primary Regulator

Breath is the most direct voluntary gateway into the autonomic nervous system. Slow, rhythmic breathing activates the **ventral vagal complex**, which supports calm attention, emotional regulation, social engagement, and cognitive clarity (Porges, 2011; Zaccaro et al., 2018).

Breathing at **4–6 cycles per minute** has been shown to:

- Increase heart rate variability
- Reduce amygdala activation
- Improve emotional stability
- Enhance working memory
- Reduce anxiety and PTSD symptoms

(Zaccaro et al., 2018; Lehrer & Gevirtz, 2014).

Breath becomes the physiological bridge between survival and growth.

From Physical Stability to Psychological Safety

Once the body begins to stabilize, psychological processes reorganize naturally. Survivors report:

- Reduced emotional volatility
- Improved impulse control
- Greater tolerance of uncertainty
- Increased reflective capacity
- More consistent self-trust

(Siegel, 2012; van der Kolk, 2014).

This is not achieved through intellectual effort alone. It emerges from **bottom-up regulation**, meaning the body leads the brain into stability.

Only when the body feels safe does deeper emotional and cognitive integration become possible.

The Somatic Basis of Post-Traumatic Growth

Post-traumatic growth depends on three bodily foundations:

1. **Regulation** – the ability to calm the nervous system
2. **Strength** – the capacity to tolerate effort and stress
3. **Embodiment** – sustained present-moment awareness

When these are restored, individuals become capable of:

- Meaning-making
- Boundary formation
- Emotional integration
- Identity reconstruction
- Purpose development

Without this somatic base, higher growth processes remain fragile and easily destabilized.

The Body as the First Site of Transformation

The body is not the obstacle to healing. It is the *instrument of healing*. Strength, posture, breath, and grounding are not preparatory exercises for later psychological work. They *are* the work.

When the body stabilizes:

- Fear loses its dominance
- Memory becomes organized
- Choice replaces compulsion
- Strength replaces helplessness

- Growth replaces survival

The restoration of embodied safety is the first reliable marker that post-traumatic growth has begun.

REFERENCES — CHAPTER 2

Critchley, H. D., & Harrison, N. A. (2013). Visceral influences on brain and behavior. *Neuron, 77*(4), 624–638. https://doi.org/10.1016/j.neuron.2013.02.008

Dishman, R. K., Berthoud, H. R., Booth, F. W., Cotman, C. W., Edgerton, V. R., Fleshner, M. R., … Zigmond, M. J. (2006). Neurobiology of exercise. *Obesity, 14*(3), 345–356. https://doi.org/10.1038/oby.2006.46

Lehrer, P., & Gevirtz, R. (2014). Heart rate variability biofeedback: How and why does it work? *Frontiers in Psychology, 5*, 756. https://doi.org/10.3389/fpsyg.2014.00756

Ogden, P., Minton, K., & Pain, C. (2006). *Trauma and the body: A sensorimotor approach to psychotherapy*. W. W. Norton & Company.

Peper, E., Lin, I., Harvey, R., & Perez, J. (2017). How posture affects memory recall and mood. *Biofeedback, 45*(2), 36–41. https://doi.org/10.5298/1081-5937-45.2.01

Porges, S. W. (2011). The polyvagal theory: Neurophysiological foundations of emotions, attachment, communication, and self-regulation. W. W. Norton & Company.

Ratey, J. J., & Loehr, J. E. (2011). The positive impact of physical activity on cognition during adulthood: A review of underlying mechanisms. *Exercise and Sport Sciences Reviews, 39*(4), 171–179. https://doi.org/10.1097/JES.0b013e31822d0a6c

Siegel, D. J. (2012). The developing mind: How relationships and the brain interact to shape who we are (2nd ed.). Guilford Press.

van der Kolk, B. A. (2014). The body keeps the score: Brain, mind, and body in the healing of trauma. Viking.

Zaccaro, A., Piarulli, A., Laurino, M., Garbella, E., Menicucci, D., Neri, B., & Gemignani, A. (2018). How breath-control can change your life: A systematic review on psychophysiological correlates of slow breathing. *Frontiers in Human Neuroscience, 12*, 353. https://doi.org/10.3389/fnhum.2018.00353

Chapter 3 - Cognitive Recovery

Discernment, Mental Clarity, and Reclaiming the Inner Narrative

Trauma does not only live in the body. It also reshapes the mind, altering how people interpret reality, evaluate threat, assign meaning, and construct identity. Survivors often describe their thinking as foggy, rigid, self-critical, pessimistic, hypervigilant, or confused. These patterns are not signs of intellectual weakness. They are the psychological footprints of survival-based learning (Beck, 1976; van der Kolk, 2014).

Trauma narrows perception. It teaches the brain to scan for danger rather than possibility. It biases interpretation toward threat, shame, and powerlessness. Over time, these cognitive adaptations solidify into internal narratives that quietly shape behavior, relationships, and life direction. Recovery therefore requires more than regulating the nervous system. It requires **reclaiming authorship of the mind itself**.

> Post-traumatic growth depends on this reclamation.

Trauma and the Rewiring of Thought

Under extreme stress, the brain prioritizes survival speed over reflective accuracy. The amygdala amplifies threat detection, while the prefrontal cortex, responsible for reasoning, judgment, and impulse control, becomes partially inhibited (LeDoux, 2012; Siegel, 2012). Memory encoding becomes fragmented, meaning becomes distorted, and learning becomes conditioned around fear rather than curiosity.

As a result, trauma survivors often develop:

- Catastrophic thinking
- Black-and-white interpretations
- Persistent self-blame
- Overgeneralization
- Emotional reasoning
- Hypervigilance to ambiguity
- Rigid belief systems

(Beck, 1976; Herman, 1992).

These thought patterns once served a protective function. They reduced uncertainty and increased vigilance. But what once helped survival now limits growth.

Conditioned Cognition and the Loss of Mental Autonomy

In many trauma histories, especially those involving abuse, coercion, neglect, or high-control environments, cognition becomes shaped by external authority rather than internal discernment. Survivors may internalize the voices of parents, institutions, religious systems, partners, or leaders who defined reality for them.

This internalization leads to:

- Chronic self-doubt
- Difficulty trusting perception
- Excessive guilt or shame
- Obedience to internalized authority
- Fear of independent thought
- Difficulty with decision-making

(Lifton, 1989; Herman, 1992).

Over time, survivors may lose psychological sovereignty, the capacity to think, evaluate, and choose freely from their own grounded center. Cognitive recovery is the process of restoring this sovereignty.

Discernment as a Core Skill of Recovery

Discernment is the ability to evaluate reality accurately without being dominated by fear, bias, or conditioning. It is not skepticism or cynicism. It is clarity.

Discernment includes the capacity to:

- Distinguish memory from present reality
- Separate fear from fact
- Recognize manipulation
- Evaluate evidence
- Detect cognitive distortions
- Sense emotional influence on thinking
- Hold nuance rather than rigid certainty

(Kahneman, 2011; Tversky & Kahneman, 1974).

Trauma weakens discernment by collapsing perception into survival binaries: safe versus dangerous, powerful versus powerless, worthy versus unworthy. Cognitive recovery restores complexity, flexibility, and choice.

Cognitive Distortions as Trauma Echoes

Cognitive distortions are not character flaws. They are learned survival interpretations. Common trauma-linked distortions include:

- **Catastrophizing** – Expecting the worst outcome
- **Personalization** – Assuming responsibility for others' behavior
- **All-or-nothing thinking** – Viewing situations as total success or failure
- **Mind-reading** – Assuming negative judgments from others
- **Emotional reasoning** – "If I feel it, it must be true"

(Beck, 1976).

These distortions persist because the nervous system remains biased toward threat. As bodily regulation improves, cognitive distortions naturally soften, but they must also be consciously examined and revised.

Reclaiming the Inner Narrative

Human identity is largely constructed through story. Psychologists refer to this as **narrative identity**, the internalized account people develop to explain who they are, where they came from, and where they are going (McAdams, 2013).

Trauma disrupts narrative continuity. Survivors may experience:

- Fragmented life stories
- Shame-dominated identity
- Confusion about values
- Disconnection between past and present
- Difficulty imagining a future

(Herman, 1992; McAdams, 2013).

Post-traumatic growth emerges when individuals consciously rewrite their narrative from one of damage to one of resilience, survival, learning, and transformation. This does not mean denying pain. It means repositioning pain within a broader context of growth.

Metacognition and the Recovery of Choice

Metacognition, the ability to observe one's own thinking, is a central mechanism of cognitive recovery (Siegel, 2012). When metacognition is strong, individuals can notice:

- "This is a trauma response."
- "This is an old belief speaking."
- "This thought is shaped by fear, not fact."
- "I have a choice in how I interpret this."

This capacity creates psychological distance from automatic reactions, restoring freedom of response. Without metacognition, individuals remain fused to conditioned thought patterns.

Meaning-Making as Cognitive Integration

Meaning-making is not philosophical abstraction. It is a neuropsychological process through which the brain organizes experience into coherence. When trauma overwhelms meaning, the psyche remains fragmented. When meaning is reconstructed, identity stabilizes (Park, 2010).

Meaning-making involves:

- Reinterpreting suffering
- Reorganizing memory
- Connecting events across time
- Assigning value to endurance
- Integrating loss into identity

Post-traumatic growth research consistently shows that **meaning-making is one of the strongest predictors of positive transformation after trauma** (Tedeschi & Calhoun, 2004; Park, 2010).

Cognitive Recovery and the Rebuilding of Trust

Trauma not only damages trust in others. It damages trust in one's own mind. Survivors may question their perceptions, minimize their intuition, or defer decision-making out of fear of being wrong.

Cognitive recovery restores:

- Self-trust
- Interpretive confidence
- Decision-making capacity
- Psychological boundaries
- Reality testing
- Discernment under pressure

This restoration allows individuals to re-enter the world without surrendering their agency.

From Fear-Based Thinking to Growth-Based Thinking

Fear-based thinking asks:

- "What will go wrong?"
- "How will I fail?"
- "Who will hurt me?"

Growth-based thinking asks:

- "What is possible now?"
- "What can I learn?"
- "Who am I becoming?"

This shift is not just positive thinking. It is **neural reorganization** that occurs when safety, regulation, and insight align (Siegel, 2012; van der Kolk, 2014).

The Cognitive Foundations of Post-Traumatic Growth

Post-traumatic growth depends on five key cognitive shifts:

1. From threat interpretation to reality-based discernment
2. From shame-based identity to coherent self-understanding
3. From conditioned thinking to psychological sovereignty
4. From fragmented memory to integrated narrative
5. From fear-based expectation to meaning-oriented anticipation

(Tedeschi & Calhoun, 2004; McAdams, 2013; Park, 2010).

When these shifts occur, individuals begin to experience not just symptom relief, but genuine psychological expansion.

The Mind as an Instrument of Growth

The mind is not the enemy of healing. It is the instrument through which meaning, purpose, values, and identity are rebuilt. When cognition is liberated from trauma-conditioned fear, it becomes the **architect of post-traumatic growth.**

As bodily regulation stabilizes and emotional integration deepens, the mind regains its natural capacity for:

- Curiosity
- Discernment
- Creativity
- Ethical reasoning

- Foresight
- Reflection
- Purpose

This cognitive freedom marks a major threshold in recovery. The survivor is no longer defined by what happened to them, but by what they now choose to become.

REFERENCES — CHAPTER 3

Beck, A. T. (1976). *Cognitive therapy and the emotional disorders*. International Universities Press.

Herman, J. L. (1992). Trauma and recovery: The aftermath of violence—from domestic abuse to political terror. Basic Books.

Kahneman, D. (2011). *Thinking, fast and slow*. Farrar, Straus and Giroux.

LeDoux, J. E. (2012). *Rethinking the emotional brain. Neuron, 73*(4), 653–676. https://doi.org/10.1016/j.neuron.2012.02.004

Lifton, R. J. (1989). Thought reform and the psychology of totalism: A study of brainwashing in China. University of North Carolina Press.

McAdams, D. P. (2013). *The redemptive self: Stories Americans live by* (Revised ed.). Oxford University Press.

Park, C. L. (2010). Making Sense of the Meaning Literature: An integrative review of meaning making and its effects on adjustment to stressful life events. *Psychological Bulletin, 136*(2), 257–301. https://doi.org/10.1037/a0018301

Siegel, D. J. (2012). The developing mind: How relationships and the brain interact to shape who we are (2nd ed.). Guilford Press.

Tedeschi, R. G., & Calhoun, L. G. (2004). Posttraumatic growth: Conceptual foundations and empirical evidence. *Psychological Inquiry, 15*(1), 1–18. https://doi.org/10.1207/s15327965pli1501_01

Tversky, A., & Kahneman, D. (1974). Judgment under uncertainty: Heuristics and biases. *Science, 185*(4157), 1124–1131. https://doi.org/10.1126/science.185.4157.1124

van der Kolk, B. A. (2014). The body keeps the score: Brain, mind, and body in the healing of trauma. Viking.

Chapter 4 - Emotional Integration

Learning to Regulate, Feel, and Transform Inner States

Trauma is fundamentally an emotional injury. While it affects the body and distorts cognition, its most persistent signature often appears in the emotional system. Survivors may struggle with emotional flooding, numbness, shame, rage, fear, grief, or sudden mood shifts that feel disconnected from present circumstances. These emotional patterns are not signs of immaturity or weakness. They are the natural byproducts of a nervous system that learned to survive under threat (Herman, 1992; van der Kolk, 2014).

Emotional integration is the process through which these fragmented affective states are gradually brought into coherence. It is not the suppression of emotion, nor the uncontrolled expression of it. It is the development of the capacity to feel without being overwhelmed, to respond without being hijacked, and to transform emotional energy into adaptive meaning.

Post-traumatic growth depends on this emotional transformation.

Trauma and the Dysregulation of Affect

Under traumatic conditions, emotional responses become shaped by survival circuits rather than reflective awareness. The amygdala becomes hypersensitive to threat, the insula amplifies bodily distress signals, and prefrontal regulation weakens (LeDoux, 2012; Siegel, 2012). As a result, emotions may emerge as:

- Sudden panic
- Explosive anger
- Persistent shame
- Emotional numbness
- Uncontrollable grief
- Chronic anxiety
- Emotional volatility

These reactions often feel confusing and disproportionate. Survivors may judge themselves harshly for their emotional responses, deepening shame and self-alienation. Yet these reactions are neurobiologically conditioned, not moral failings (van der Kolk, 2014).

Emotion as a Constructed Neurophysiological Process

Modern affective neuroscience shows that emotions are not fixed entities that simply "happen." They are **constructed experiences**, built from:

- Autonomic nervous system states
- Interoceptive sensations
- Memory
- Cognitive interpretation
- Social context

(Barrett, 2017).

This means emotions are **malleable**, not permanent. The emotional brain is plastic. With new bodily regulation, new cognitive frames, and new relational experiences, emotional responses reorganize. This plasticity forms the biological foundation of emotional integration and post-traumatic growth.

From Emotional Suppression to Emotional Capacity

Many trauma survivors learned early that emotional expression was unsafe, punished, ignored, or exploited. As a result, they may default to:

- Emotional suppression
- Emotional minimization
- Intellectualization
- Numbing behaviors
- Compulsive distraction
- Addictive regulation strategies

(Herman, 1992; van der Kolk, 2014).

While these strategies once served survival, they now restrict emotional capacity. Growth requires not the elimination of emotion, but the expansion of the nervous system's ability to tolerate emotional intensity without destabilization.

This capacity develops gradually through regulation, not through force.

Emotional Regulation as a Learned Skill

Emotional regulation is not a personality trait. It is a **trainable neurobiological capacity** that depends on vagal tone, prefrontal engagement, and interoceptive awareness (Porges, 2011; Siegel, 2012).

Regulation allows individuals to:

- Pause before reacting
- Stay present with difficult feelings
- Soften physiological arousal
- Prevent emotional escalation
- Maintain relational connection under stress
- Choose responses consciously

Without regulation, emotions dominate behavior. With regulation, emotions inform behavior without controlling it.

The Role of the Body in Emotional Integration

Because emotion arises first as bodily sensation, emotional integration must proceed from the body upward. Key somatic contributors include:

- Breath rhythm
- Postural stability
- Muscle tone
- Visceral sensation
- Heart rate variability
- Ground contact

(Porges, 2011; Zaccaro et al., 2018).

When the body stabilizes, emotional reactivity decreases. When the body remains dysregulated, no amount of insight prevents emotional overwhelm. Emotional integration therefore remains tightly linked to the somatic foundation established in Chapter 2.

Shame as a Central Trauma Emotion

Among all trauma-related emotions, shame is often the most corrosive. Shame is not guilt for behavior. It is the belief that the self is fundamentally defective. Research shows that shame strongly predicts depression, addiction, dissociation, and relational dysfunction (Tangney & Dearing, 2002).

Trauma often produces shame through:

- Victim-blaming
- Chronic invalidation

- Powerlessness
- Humiliation
- Betrayal
- Moral injury

Emotional integration requires the systematic dismantling of shame through:

- Accurate attribution of responsibility
- Self-compassion
- Meaning-making
- Relational safety
- Restoration of dignity

(Neff, 2011; Herman, 1992).

Without addressing shame, post-traumatic growth remains blocked.

Anger, Grief, and Fear as Adaptive Signals

Trauma-related emotions often become pathologized. Yet anger, grief, and fear all serve adaptive functions:

- **Fear** signals threat and guides boundary formation
- **Anger** signals violation and mobilizes self-protection
- **Grief** signals loss and reorganizes attachment

When these emotions are suppressed or distorted, they become chronic. When they are felt, regulated, and integrated, they guide growth.

Emotional integration does not ask, "How do I get rid of this emotion?" It asks, "What is this emotion trying to protect, restore, or reveal?"

Psychological Flexibility and Emotional Maturity

Psychological flexibility refers to the ability to experience emotions without avoidance or over-identification, while continuing to act in alignment with values (Kashdan & Rottenberg, 2010). It is one of the strongest predictors of long-term mental health.

Emotionally mature individuals can:

- Feel deeply without collapsing

- Express emotion without aggression
- Tolerate ambivalence
- Sit with uncertainty
- Experience sorrow without despair
- Experience anger without violence

Trauma narrows this flexibility. Emotional integration restores it.

Compassion as an Outcome of Emotional Integration

Compassion is not a moral command. It is a neurobiological outcome of emotional regulation and integration. When threat-based reactivity softens, the brain reopens social engagement systems, empathy, and relational attunement (Porges, 2011; Leiberg et al., 2011).

Compassion arises naturally when individuals:

- Can feel without being overwhelmed
- Can regulate without suppressing
- Can witness suffering without dissociating
- Can remain present without fear

This is one of the most consistent markers of post-traumatic growth (Tedeschi & Calhoun, 2018).

Emotional Transformation and Post-Traumatic Growth

Post-traumatic growth requires not emotional avoidance, but **emotional reorganization**. Survivors who experience PTG report:

- Greater emotional depth
- Increased empathy
- Expanded emotional range
- Enhanced relational intimacy
- Stronger emotional boundaries
- Greater tolerance of suffering in self and others

(Tedeschi & Calhoun, 2004, 2018).

This transformation occurs because the emotional system is no longer organized around survival alone. It becomes organized around meaning, values, and connection.

From Emotional Reactivity to Emotional Wisdom

Emotional wisdom is not the absence of emotion. It is the ability to:

- Recognize emotional signals accurately
- Regulate emotional intensity
- Interpret emotional meaning
- Integrate emotion with cognition
- Translate emotion into ethical action

When emotional integration is achieved, feelings no longer dictate identity or behavior. They become informative signals within a coherent self-system.

Emotional Integration as the Bridge Between Survival and Growth

The emotional system sits at the center of the trauma recovery process. The body provides stability. The mind provides meaning. But emotion provides movement between the two. It is the bridge through which sensation becomes meaning and meaning becomes relationship.

Until emotion is integrated, growth remains intellectual. When emotion is integrated, growth becomes embodied and relational.

This marks the transition from symptom management to post-traumatic growth.

REFERENCES — CHAPTER 4

Barrett, L. F. (2017). *How emotions are made: The secret life of the brain*. Houghton Mifflin Harcourt.

Herman, J. L. (1992). Trauma and recovery: The aftermath of violence—from domestic abuse to political terror. Basic Books.

Kashdan, T. B., & Rottenberg, J. (2010). Psychological flexibility as a fundamental aspect of health. *Clinical Psychology Review, 30*(7), 865–878.
https://doi.org/10.1016/j.cpr.2010.03.001

LeDoux, J. E. (2012). *Rethinking the emotional brain. Neuron, 73*(4), 653–676.
https://doi.org/10.1016/j.neuron.2012.02.004

Leiberg, S., Klimecki, O., & Singer, T. (2011). Short-term compassion training increases prosocial behavior in a newly developed prosocial game. *PloS one*, *6*(3), e17798. https://doi.org/10.1371/journal.pone.0017798

Neff, K. D. (2011). Self-compassion: The proven power of being kind to yourself. William Morrow.

Porges, S. W. (2011). The polyvagal theory: Neurophysiological foundations of emotions, attachment, communication, and self-regulation. W. W. Norton & Company.

Siegel, D. J. (2012). The developing mind: How relationships and the brain interact to shape who we are (2nd ed.). Guilford Press.

Tangney, J. P., & Dearing, R. L. (2002). *Shame and guilt*. Guilford Press.

Tedeschi, R. G., & Calhoun, L. G. (2004). Posttraumatic growth: Conceptual foundations and empirical evidence. *Psychological Inquiry, 15*(1), 1–18. https://doi.org/10.1207/s15327965pli1501_01

Tedeschi, R. G., & Calhoun, L. G. (2018). Posttraumatic growth: Theory, research, and applications. Routledge.

van der Kolk, B. A. (2014). The body keeps the score: Brain, mind, and body in the healing of trauma. Viking.

Zaccaro, A., Piarulli, A., Laurino, M., Garbella, E., Menicucci, D., Neri, B., & Gemignani, A. (2018). How breath-control can change your life: A systematic review on psychophysiological correlates of slow breathing. *Frontiers in Human Neuroscience, 12*, 353. https://doi.org/10.3389/fnhum.2018.00353

Part II — The Physiology of Healing and Self-Regulation

Chapter 5 - Breath, Posture, and Nervous System Regulation in Post-Traumatic Growth

Breath and posture are not merely mechanical functions of the body. They are the most direct and reliable gateways into the autonomic nervous system, the system that governs survival, emotional regulation, attention, digestion, cardiovascular function, immune response, and social engagement. Trauma disrupts these systems at their root. As a result, breath becomes restricted, posture becomes defensive, and nervous system regulation becomes unstable (Porges, 2011; van der Kolk, 2014).

Post-traumatic growth requires not only emotional insight and cognitive clarity, but also physiological mastery. When breath and posture are restored, the nervous system regains its capacity for flexibility, resilience, and coherent response. This chapter explores how breath and posture operate as primary tools of nervous system rehabilitation and transformation after trauma.

The Autonomic Nervous System and Trauma

The autonomic nervous system operates through two primary branches:

- **The sympathetic system**, responsible for mobilization (fight or flight)
- **The parasympathetic system**, responsible for restoration (rest, digestion, recovery) – **(see appendix A)**

Within the parasympathetic system, the ventral vagal pathway supports calm presence, emotional regulation, social connection, and cognitive clarity, while the dorsal vagal pathway mediates shutdown, collapse, and dissociation under overwhelming threat (Porges, 2011).

Trauma dysregulates these systems. Survivors often become stuck in:

- **Chronic sympathetic activation** (anxiety, agitation, hypervigilance)
- **Chronic dorsal vagal dominance** (numbness, depression, fatigue, dissociation)

Nervous system mastery is the process of restoring **flexible oscillation** between activation and recovery. Breath and posture are the most efficient points of entry into this process.

Breath as the Primary Regulator of Autonomic State

Breathing is unique among physiological functions because it is both automatic and voluntarily controllable. This makes it the most accessible tool for regulating autonomic arousal (Zaccaro et al., 2018).

Slow, rhythmic breathing directly:

- Activates the ventral vagal complex
- Reduces amygdala hyperreactivity
- Increases heart-rate variability (HRV)
- Stabilizes emotional intensity
- Improves executive functioning
- Enhances interoceptive awareness

(Lehrer & Gevirtz, 2014; Porges, 2011; Zaccaro et al., 2018).

Breathing at approximately **4–6 cycles per minute** has been shown to produce the strongest improvements in vagal tone and emotional regulation. This breathing rhythm becomes the physiological signature of safety within the body. **(see appendix B – Box Breathing)**

Trauma, Breath Restriction, and Threat Signaling

Trauma survivors rarely breathe freely. Common patterns include:

- Shallow chest breathing
- Chronic breath holding
- Irregular rhythm
- Excessive sighing
- Restricted exhalation

These patterns maintain continuous threat signaling to the brain. Restricted exhalation, in particular, sustains sympathetic arousal and prevents full parasympathetic recovery (Zaccaro et al., 2018).

Restoring healthy breathing restores:

- Emotional stability
- Cognitive clarity
- Sleep regulation
- Stress tolerance
- Interpersonal regulation

Breath becomes the physiological language of safety.

BREATH, POSTURE, & AUTONOMIC REGULATION

BREATH CONTROL
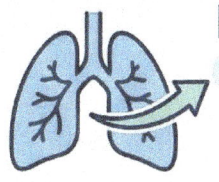
- Deep Diaphragmatic Breathing
- Extended Exhale
- Vagus Nerve Stimulation

PHYSICAL POSTURE
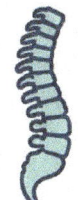 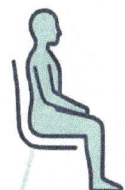
- Upright Alignment
- Chest Open/Spine Neutral
- Reduced Muscular Tension

AUTONOMIC NERVOUS SYSTEM REGULATION
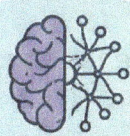

SYNERGISTIC REGULATION

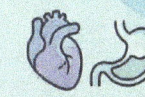
PARASYMPATHETIC ACTIVATION
(Rest & Digest, Calm)

SYMPATHETIC MODULATION
(Stress Response, Alertness)

OVERALL WELL-BEING & HOMEOSTASIS
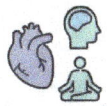
- Reduced Chronic Stress
- Improved Emotional Balance
- Enhanced Resilience
- Optimized Physiological Function

Posture as a Nervous System Signal

Posture is a continuous message sent from the body to the brain. Upright, supported posture enhances:

- Prefrontal engagement
- Emotional regulation
- Memory recall
- Self-confidence
- Mood stability

Collapsed or rigid posture amplifies:

- Fear-based cognition
- Rumination
- Depression
- Helplessness
- Emotional reactivity

(Peper et al., 2016; Siegel, 2012).

Trauma conditions the body toward defensive architecture. Postural restoration is therefore not cosmetic. It is a neurological intervention.

Postural Patterns Common in Trauma

Trauma-associated posture often includes:

- Forward head carriage
- Rounded shoulders
- Compressed chest
- Locked jaw
- Guarded abdomen
- Collapsed stance or rigid stiffness

These patterns reflect chronic sympathetic activation or dorsal vagal collapse. They reduce oxygen exchange, restrict vagal signaling, impair balance, and compromise emotional regulation.

Corrective postural work reverses these effects by restoring:

- Spinal alignment
- Diaphragmatic movement

- Stable base of support
- Balanced muscle tone

(Peper et al., 2016; Ogden et al., 2006).

The Breath - Posture - Emotion Triad

Breath, posture, and emotion form a tightly coupled triad:

- Posture shapes breathing
- Breathing shapes emotion
- Emotion shapes cognition
- Cognition reinforces posture

(Siegel, 2012; Porges, 2011).

When one element shifts, the entire system reorganizes. This is why bottom-up interventions are so effective in trauma recovery. A person does not need to "convince" themselves they are safe. **Their body learns safety through direct physiological experience.**

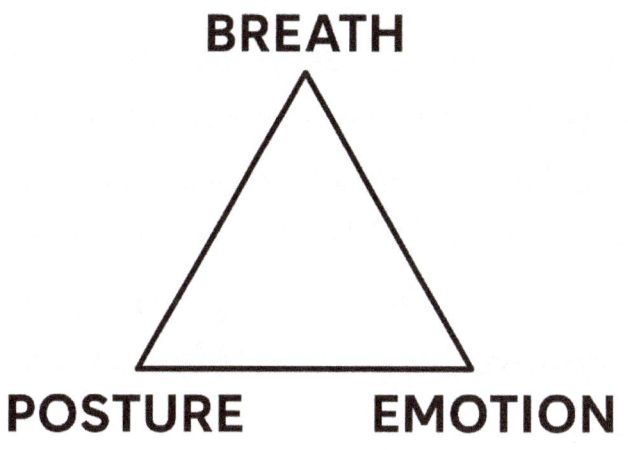

Nervous System Mastery as a Trainable Capacity

Nervous system regulation is not an inborn talent. It is a trainable biological skill. Through consistent breath training, posture correction, and slow movement, individuals strengthen:

- Vagal tone
- Stress tolerance
- Emotional containment
- Attentional stability
- Impulse control
- Social engagement capacity

(Porges, 2011; Lehrer & Gevirtz, 2014; Zaccaro et al., 2018).

Over time, the nervous system becomes less reactive and more responsive. This shift marks a major threshold in post-traumatic growth.

Physiological Containment and Emotional Safety

Containment refers to the body's ability to hold emotional intensity without fragmentation or overwhelm. It depends on:

- Postural stability
- Breath depth
- Core muscular tone
- Ground contact
- Autonomic balance

When containment is weak, emotions overflow. When containment is strong, emotions can be felt, explored, and integrated without destabilization.

This capacity is essential for advanced stages of emotional integration, identity reconstruction, and relational healing.

Breath Training and Cognitive Function

Breath regulation does not only affect emotion. It directly enhances cognitive performance by:

- Increasing oxygen delivery
- Improving prefrontal cortex activation
- Reducing limbic interference
- Enhancing attention and working memory

(Zaccaro et al., 2018; Lehrer & Gevirtz, 2014).

As cognitive clarity improves, discernment and narrative reconstruction (Chapter 3) become more accessible and stable.

Social Regulation and the Nervous System

The ventral vagal system governs not only personal calm, but also **relational engagement**. When breath and posture stabilize, individuals naturally exhibit:

- Softer facial expression
- Clearer vocal tone
- Increased eye contact
- Greater emotional availability
- Reduced defensiveness

(Porges, 2011; Siegel, 2012).

This shift supports relational repair and attachment healing, which are critical components of post-traumatic growth.

Applied Regulation Practice: Breath, Posture, and Nervous System Stabilization

This chapter translates the physiology of breath and posture into clear, trauma-informed mechanisms for **nervous system regulation**, **emotional stability**, and **post-traumatic growth (PTG)**. Recovery is not achieved through insight alone. It is achieved through the repeated restoration of safety, coherence, and agency within the body. Breath and posture provide two of the most reliable, accessible, and evidence-supported entry points into that process.

The nervous system does not distinguish between psychological threats and physical threats. It responds to **signals of safety or danger**, and breath and posture are among the most powerful sources of those signals. When they are trained intentionally, they become tools not only for symptom relief, but for long-term recalibration of stress response, emotional regulation, and self-directed recovery.

1. Breath as a Primary Regulator of the Nervous System

Breathing is unique among physiological functions because it is both automatic and voluntary (Lehrer & Gevirtz, 2014; Zaccaro et al., 2018). This dual nature allows breath to serve as a direct access point to the autonomic nervous system. In trauma, breathing commonly becomes shallow, rapid, irregular, or held. These patterns reinforce sympathetic arousal, hypervigilance, panic, and emotional volatility.

Slow, rhythmical breathing exerts its regulatory effects through vagal signaling, baroreflex sensitivity, and heart-rate variability (Porges, 2011; Zaccaro et al., 2018). its regulatory effects through vagal signaling, baroreflex sensitivity, and heart-rate variability. When the breath is slowed, extended, and stabilized, particularly through prolonged exhalation, parasympathetic activity increases and stress hormones decline. This shift supports cognitive clarity, emotional steadiness, and physiological safety.

Breath regulation also improves **interoceptive awareness**, the capacity to perceive internal bodily states. Trauma often disrupts this awareness, leading individuals to feel either overwhelmed by bodily sensations or disconnected from them altogether. Restoring interoception through breath training supports emotional literacy, boundary awareness, and self-regulation.

Clinical Effects of Regulated Breathing

- Reduction in anxiety and panic symptoms
- Improved emotional regulation
- Enhanced attentional control
- Stabilization of autonomic arousal
- Improved sleep onset and sleep continuity

2. Posture as a Modulator of Emotion and Cognition

Posture is not a neutral mechanical state; it continuously influences emotion and cognition through proprioceptive signaling (Peper et al., 2016). It is a continuous stream of neurological information sent from the body to the brain. Chronic trauma patterns often leave the body in collapsed, guarded, asymmetrical, or rigid positions that silently reinforce fear, shame, helplessness, and vigilance.

Upright, balanced posture sends a different message through proprioceptive and vestibular pathways. It supports respiratory efficiency, vagal tone, and frontal-limbic regulation. Changes in posture alone can measurably influence emotional state, confidence, memory recall, and stress perception.

Postural correction in trauma recovery is not about rigid "good posture." It is about restoring **dynamic alignment,** the capacity to remain upright, grounded, and relaxed at the same time. This balance allows the nervous system to remain responsive without becoming defensive.

Common Trauma-Associated Postural Patterns

- Forward head and rounded shoulders
- Collapsed chest and shallow breathing
- Asymmetrical weight bearing
- Chronic jaw, neck, or shoulder tension

These patterns reinforce the internal narrative of threat. Postural retraining gently interrupts that narrative at the physiological level.

3. Polyvagal Regulation and Autonomic State Shifting

The autonomic nervous system operates through two primary branches: **sympathetic activation** (mobilization) and **parasympathetic regulation** (restoration). Trauma locks many individuals into cycles of hyperarousal or shutdown. Breath and posture function as autonomic levers that help shift these states safely.

Slow nasal breathing, extended exhalation, upright posture, and grounded stance all increase vagal signaling. This shift promotes:

- Improved social engagement capacity
- Enhanced emotional buffering
- Reduced defensive reactivity
- Greater tolerance for stress without collapse

Post-traumatic growth requires more than symptom reduction. It requires the restoration of **state flexibility,** the capacity to move between activation and rest without becoming trapped in either.

4. Trauma, Somatic Patterning, and Recovery

Trauma is stored not only as memory, but as motor, breath, and postural pattern (van der Kolk, 2014; Ogden et al., 2006)., but as **motor pattern, breath pattern, and postural pattern**. These somatic imprints operate below conscious awareness yet strongly influence emotion, perception, and behavior. Attempts to "think" one's way out of trauma often fail because the body continues to broadcast threat signals even when the mind understands safety.

Somatic regulation reverses this sequence. When breath slows and posture reorganizes, the brain receives new sensory information that supports safety and coherence. Over time, repeated somatic stabilization alters limbic conditioning and reduces the baseline expectation of danger.

Recovery is therefore not a single event. It is the accumulation of thousands of small regulatory repetitions that gradually shift the nervous system out of survival mode and into adaptive engagement.

5. Daily Practices for Nervous System Mastery

The following practices are designed for **daily implementation**. Their power lies not in intensity, but in consistency. Short, frequent repetitions are neurologically superior to rare, dramatic efforts. **(see appendices for color detailed graphics on these practices)**

1. Coherent Breathing

- Inhale 4–5 seconds
- Exhale 5–6 seconds
- Practice 5 minutes, 2–3 times per day

2. Physiological Sigh

- Inhale through the nose
- Brief second sniff
- Long slow exhale through the mouth
- Repeat 3–5 cycles

3. Grounded Standing

- Feet hip-width
- Knees soft
- Spine vertical
- Jaw unclenched
- Breath slowly and through the nose
- 2–5 minutes

4. Postural Reset Sequence

- Gentle chin tuck
- Shoulder roll back and down
- Rib cage stacked over pelvis
- Weight balanced evenly

5. Somatic Scanning

- Slow attention through feet, legs, pelvis, spine, shoulders, neck, jaw
- Identify tension without forcing release

These practices restore **neurological authorship**, where one gains the capacity to influence one's own state rather than remain at the mercy of automatic stress reactions.

6. Nervous System Mastery and Post-Traumatic Growth

Post-traumatic growth is not only a psychological transformation. It is a biological recalibration. Breath and posture provide the most reliable daily access to that recalibration because they:

- Restore autonomic balance

- Strengthen emotional regulation
- Increase stress tolerance
- Improve self-trust
- Support identity reconstruction

Through these mechanisms, the individual moves from reactivity to responsiveness, from collapse to coherence, and from survival mode into sustainable engagement with life.

Breath and posture do not merely manage symptoms. They re-educate the nervous system toward safety, agency, and growth.

From Physiological Survival to Physiological Growth

Before recovery, the body is organized around **survival**. After regulation is restored, the body reorganizes around **growth**. This transition is marked by:

- Reduced baseline anxiety
- Improved sleep
- Stable digestion
- Increased energy
- Enhanced emotional presence
- Greater psychological resilience

These are not abstract benefits. They reflect real neurophysiological transformation.

Nervous System Mastery as a Cornerstone of Post-Traumatic Growth

Without nervous system mastery, trauma recovery remains fragile and unstable. With it, higher capacities emerge naturally:

- Meaning-making
- Boundary formation
- Emotional integration
- Identity reconstruction
- Purpose development
- Compassion
- Relational maturity

Breath and posture do not replace psychological work. They make psychological work possible and sustainable.

The Body as the Gateway to Growth

Post-traumatic growth begins not with insight, but with **stability**. The body must learn that the present is not the past. Breath teaches this. Posture teaches this. Nervous system mastery embodies this truth at a cellular level.

When the body becomes safe, the mind becomes clear.
When the mind becomes clear, the heart becomes open.
When the heart becomes open, growth becomes inevitable.

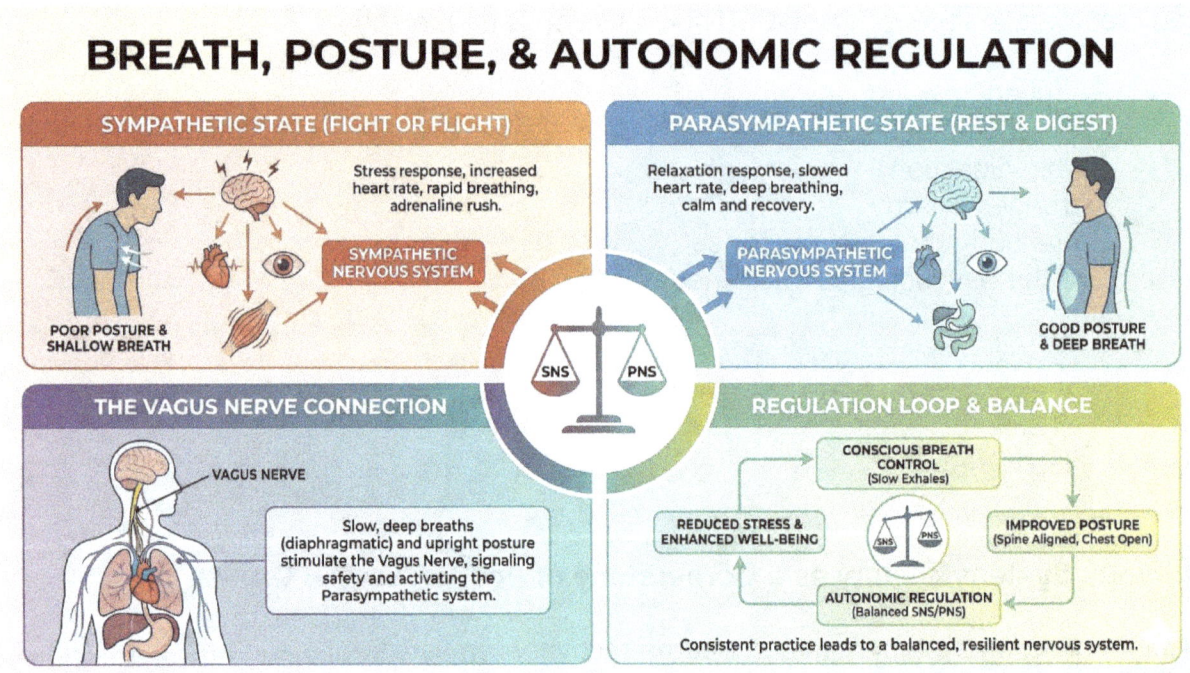

REFERENCES — CHAPTER 5

Lehrer, P. M., & Gevirtz, R. (2014). Heart rate variability biofeedback: How and why does it work? *Frontiers in Psychology, 5*, 756. https://doi.org/10.3389/fpsyg.2014.00756

Ogden, P., Minton, K., & Pain, C. (2006). *Trauma and the body: A sensorimotor approach to psychotherapy*. W. W. Norton & Company.

Peper, E., Lin, I. M., Harvey, R., & Perez, J. (2016). How posture affects memory recall and mood. *Biofeedback, 44*(1), 36–41. https://doi.org/10.5298/1081-5937-44.1.02

Porges, S. W. (2011). The polyvagal theory: Neurophysiological foundations of emotions, attachment, communication, and self-regulation. W. W. Norton & Company.

Siegel, D. J. (2012). The developing mind: How relationships and the brain interact to shape who we are (2nd ed.). Guilford Press.

van der Kolk, B. A. (2014). The body keeps the score: Brain, mind, and body in the healing of trauma. Viking.

Zaccaro, A., Piarulli, A., Laurino, M., Garbella, E., Menicucci, D., Neri, B., & Gemignani, A. (2018). How breath-control can change your life: A systematic review on psychophysiological correlates of slow breathing. *Frontiers in Human Neuroscience, 12*, 353. https://doi.org/10.3389/fnhum.2018.00353

Chapter 6 - Practical Methods of Emotional and Physiological Self-Regulation

Trauma recovery requires more than understanding the body and mind. It requires active self-regulation skills that can stabilize the nervous system, reduce emotional overwhelm, and restore a sense of internal control. Self-regulation is the bridge between insight and transformation. It allows survivors to navigate intense emotions, intrusive memories, relational triggers, and stress without losing stability (Siegel, 2012; Porges, 2011).

Self-regulation skills are not innate. They are trainable capacities that strengthen neural pathways associated with safety, agency, and emotional resilience. These methods form the core of nervous system rehabilitation and lay the groundwork for deeper psychological work.

Why Self-Regulation Is Essential for Post-Traumatic Growth

Trauma disrupts the ability to modulate arousal. Survivors often oscillate between:

- **Hyperarousal** — anxiety, panic, anger, impulsiveness, hypervigilance
- **Hypoarousal** — numbness, collapse, dissociation, fatigue

These states interfere with cognition, emotion regulation, decision-making, and relationships (van der Kolk, 2014). Without reliable self-regulation tools, survivors may remain reactive rather than responsive.

Self-regulation empowers individuals to:

- Reduce physiological distress
- Re-engage the prefrontal cortex
- Maintain emotional stability
- Reduce avoidance
- Tolerate discomfort
- Build trust in their own internal capacity

This shift is foundational for post-traumatic growth, which depends on the ability to engage meaning-making, relational repair, and identity reconstruction from a grounded, regulated state (Tedeschi & Calhoun, 2018).

I. Breath-Based Regulation

Breath remains the most immediate and versatile regulation tool. Different breathing patterns produce distinct effects on the autonomic nervous system (Zaccaro et al., 2018). **(see appendices for color detailed graphics on these practices)**

1. Coherent Breathing (4–6 Breaths Per Minute)

Purpose: Activate the ventral vagal system; reduce anxiety; stabilize attention
Method:

- Inhale through the nose for ~5 seconds
- Exhale for ~5 seconds
- Continue for 3–10 minutes

This pattern increases heart-rate variability (HRV), improves emotional control, and reduces limbic reactivity (Lehrer & Gevirtz, 2014). It is one of the most evidence-based breath practices for trauma recovery.

2. Extended Exhalation Breathing

Purpose: Reduce sympathetic arousal; exit fight-or-flight
Method:

- Inhale naturally
- Exhale slowly for twice as long (e.g., inhale 4 seconds, exhale 8 seconds)

Prolonged exhalation engages the parasympathetic system and is particularly effective for panic and agitation (Porges, 2011).

3. Box Breathing

Purpose: Increase cognitive control; stabilize overwhelmed states
Method:

- Inhale 4 seconds
- Hold 4 seconds
- Exhale 4 seconds
- Hold 4 seconds

Used widely in high-stress populations (e.g., military, emergency response), this pattern increases prefrontal cortex activation and attention stability (Norelli et al., 2023). **(see appendix B – Box Breathing)**

II. Somatic Grounding Techniques

Grounding shifts awareness from overwhelming internal states to the immediate environment or body sensations. It is one of the most effective interventions for dissociation, rumination, and emotional flooding (Ogden et al., 2006).

4. The 5-4-3-2-1 Sensory Method

Purpose: Reduce dissociation and panic
Grounding through sensory engagement:

- 5 things you can see
- 4 you can touch
- 3 you can hear
- 2 you can smell
- 1 you can taste

This interrupts dissociative spirals and reorients attention to the present moment.

5. Weighted Grounding (Feet + Pressure)

Purpose: Reduce dorsal vagal shutdown; restore bodily presence
Method:

- Stand with feet hip-width
- Press feet lightly into the floor
- Notice weight, temperature, and contact

This technique increases somatosensory feedback and reduces dissociative drift (Ogden et al., 2006).

6. Orienting Response Training

Purpose: Teach the nervous system that the environment is safe
Method:

- Look slowly around the room
- Let the eyes land where they feel drawn
- Notice colors, textures, shapes
- Breathe as you orient

This method taps into primal threat-assessment circuitry but redirects it toward safety recognition (Porges, 2011).

III. Postural and Movement-Based Regulation

Posture and slow, intentional movement reorganize emotional and physiological states (Peper et al., 2016). Trauma survivors often carry defensive postures that maintain chronic arousal or collapse.

7. Postural Reset: Lengthen the Spine, Open the Chest

Purpose: Reduce depressive affect; increase cognitive engagement
Correcting posture increases vagal tone and reduces negative affect (Peper et al., 2016).
Method:

- Imagine a string lifting the crown of the head
- Relax shoulders
- Expand the sternum slightly
- Breathe into the ribcage

8. Slow, Rhythmic Movement (Walking, Swaying, Weight-Shifting)

Purpose: Restore autonomic flexibility; reduce sympathetic charge
Slow movement entrains the breath and reduces hyperarousal (Toth et al., 2023).

9. Tremoring / Shaking Release

Purpose: Discharge excess sympathetic energy
Mild voluntary shaking activates natural stress-release pathways and decreases muscular defense patterns (Berceli & Napoli, 2006).

IV. Cognitive-Somatic Integration Techniques

Trauma recovery is most efficient when cognitive awareness and somatic experience work together.

10. Name the State ("Labeling the Experience")

Purpose: Reduce amygdala activation
Affective labeling, or putting words to emotion, reduces limbic activity and strengthens prefrontal control (Lieberman et al., 2007).
Examples:

- "I feel anxious."
- "My chest is tight."
- "This is a trauma memory, not the present."

11. Pendulation (Titrated Attention)

Purpose: Build emotional tolerance without overwhelming.
Developed by somatic trauma practitioners, pendulation involves:

- Focusing briefly on distress
- Then shifting to a neutral or positive sensation
- Repeating gently

This prevents over-activation and increases regulation (Ogden et al., 2006).

12. Self-Compassionate Reappraisal

Purpose: Reduce shame; stabilize emotional interpretation
Self-compassion reduces cortisol, shame, and self-criticism while increasing resilience

(Neff, 2011).
Example:

- "I am struggling, but I am not failing."
- "This response makes sense given my history."

V. Building a Personalized Regulation Toolkit

No single method works for everyone. Survivors benefit most from an individualized toolkit that addresses:

- Hyperarousal
- Hypoarousal
- Emotional flooding
- Dissociation
- Cognitive overwhelm
- Relational triggers

Developing a toolkit restores **agency**, one of the central features of post-traumatic growth (Tedeschi & Calhoun, 2018).

The goal is not to eliminate emotional discomfort but to remain stable enough to grow.

VI. Self-Regulation as Identity Reconstruction

Consistent regulation practice teaches survivors:

- "My body is not my enemy."
- "I can influence my internal state."
- "I am capable of stability."
- "I can return to myself after being triggered."

This shifts identity from helplessness to capability, from chaos to coherence.

Emotional and physiological mastery is not a secondary aspect of recovery, but rather it is a defining milestone of post-traumatic growth.

REFERENCES — CHAPTER 6

Berceli, D., & Napoli, M. (2006). A proposal for a Mindfulness-Based Trauma Prevention Program for social work professionals. *Complementary Health Practice Review, 11*(3), 153–165. https://doi.org/10.1177/1533210106297989

Lieberman, M. D., Eisenberger, N. I., Crockett, M. J., et al. (2007). Putting feelings into words: Affect labeling disrupts amygdala activity. *Psychological Science, 18*(5), 421–428. https://doi.org/10.1111/j.1467-9280.2007.01916.x

Neff, K. D. (2011). Self-compassion: The proven power of being kind to yourself. William Morrow.

Norelli, S. K., Long, A., & Krepps, J. M. (2023, August 28). *Relaxation techniques*. StatPearls - NCBI Bookshelf. https://www.ncbi.nlm.nih.gov/books/NBK513238/

Ogden, P., Minton, K., & Pain, C. (2006). *Trauma and the body: A sensorimotor approach to psychotherapy*. W. W. Norton & Company.

Peper, E., Lin, I. M., Harvey, R., & Perez, J. (2016). How posture affects memory recall and mood. *Biofeedback, 44*(1), 36–41. https://doi.org/10.5298/1081-5937-44.1.02

Porges, S. W. (2011). The polyvagal theory: Neurophysiological foundations of emotions, attachment, communication, and self-regulation. W. W. Norton & Company.

Siegel, D. J. (2012). The developing mind: How relationships and the brain interact to shape who we are (2nd ed.). Guilford Press.

Tedeschi, R. G., & Calhoun, L. G. (2018). Posttraumatic growth: Theory, research, and applications. Routledge.

Toth, E. E., Ihász, F., Ruíz-Barquín, R., & Szabo, A. (2023). Physical Activity and Psychological Resilience in Older Adults: A Systematic Review of the Literature. *Journal of aging and physical activity, 32*(2), 276–286. https://doi.org/10.1123/japa.2022-0427

van der Kolk, B. A. (2014). The body keeps the score: Brain, mind, and body in the healing of trauma. Viking.

Zaccaro, A., Piarulli, A., Laurino, M., Garbella, E., Menicucci, D., Neri, B., & Gemignani, A. (2018). How breath-control can change your life: A systematic review on psychophysiological correlates of slow breathing. *Frontiers in Human Neuroscience, 12*, 353. https://doi.org/10.3389/fnhum.2018.00353

Chapter 7 - Rewiring the Stress Response

Trauma conditions the nervous system to perceive stress as danger. As a result, survivors often become either hyperreactive to challenge or avoiding all forms of discomfort. While this response once served survival, it eventually narrows life, restricts growth, and reinforces fear-based identity. Post-traumatic growth requires not only safety and regulation, but the **gradual restoration of the nervous system's capacity to tolerate, recover from, and ultimately grow through stress** (Dienstbier, 1989; Southwick et al., 2014).

This process is known as stress inoculation or controlled exposure to manageable challenges. When stress is introduced in measured, time-limited, and voluntary ways, it strengthens rather than overwhelms the nervous system. Through repeated cycles of challenge and recovery, the stress response becomes rewired from fragility to resilience.

Trauma, Avoidance, and the Narrowing of Capacity

After trauma, the nervous system learns that arousal equals danger. This produces powerful avoidance patterns, including:

- Avoidance of emotional intensity
- Avoidance of physical exertion
- Avoidance of confrontation
- Avoidance of novelty
- Avoidance of uncertainty

These patterns shrink the nervous system's tolerance window and reinforce helplessness (Herman, 1992; van der Kolk, 2014). Avoidance reduces short-term distress but increases long-term vulnerability. Each avoided challenge silently teaches the brain: "I cannot tolerate this."

Post-traumatic growth requires reversing this learning through graduated stress exposure that remains within the individual's window of tolerance (Siegel, 2012).

The Biology of Stress Adaptation

Not all stress is harmful. Research in psychophysiology shows that **intermittent, moderate stress strengthens regulatory systems**, while chronic, uncontrollable stress degrades them. This adaptive principle is known as **hormesis** (Dienstbier, 1989; McEwen & Wingfield, 2003).

Positive adaptations to controlled stress include:

- Increased autonomic flexibility
- Improved cortisol regulation
- Enhanced emotional containment
- Increased pain tolerance
- Improved immune function
- Greater psychological endurance

The same nervous system that was once overwhelmed by trauma can, under the right conditions, be retrained to grow stronger through challenge.

From Survival Arousal to Adaptive Arousal

Trauma generates **non-voluntary arousal** accompanied by helplessness and threat. In contrast, controlled discomfort produces **voluntary arousal** accompanied by agency and containment. This distinction is critical.

Adaptive arousal is characterized by:

- Choice
- Predictability
- Containment
- Recovery
- Meaning

When these conditions are present, stress no longer imprints trauma. It imprints **resilience** (Dienstbier, 1989; Southwick et al., 2014).

Stress Inoculation and the Window of Tolerance

The **window of tolerance** refers to the optimal arousal zone in which individuals can engage stress without becoming hyperaroused or dissociated (Siegel, 2012).

- Above the window → panic, rage, shutdown
- Below the window → numbness, disengagement
- Inside the window → learning, strength, integration

Effective resilience training always occurs inside the window, then gradually expands it. This prevents re-traumatization while steadily increasing capacity.

Eustress: When Stress Builds Strength Instead of Breaking It

Not all stress is harmful. While chronic, overwhelming stress (*distress*) erodes health and impairs recovery, a different category of stress is **eustress,** and it plays a critical role in human adaptation, learning, and post-traumatic growth. Eustress refers to **moderate, time-limited, and meaningful challenge** that activates physiological arousal in ways that strengthen resilience rather than deplete it.

From a biological perspective, eustress operates through the same stress-response systems as distress, yet with a fundamentally different outcome. When arousal is predictable, controllable, and paired with recovery, the nervous system adapts rather than deteriorates. This adaptive process is reflected in improved autonomic flexibility, enhanced cardiovascular regulation, and strengthened stress tolerance, mechanisms closely related to **allostasis** and physiological toughness (Dienstbier, 1989; McEwen & Wingfield, 2003).

Eustress is evident in domains such as:

- **Physical training and exercise**, where controlled strain produces neurobiological and cognitive benefits (Dishman et al., 2006; Ratey & Loehr, 2011),
- **Exposure-based therapies**, where gradual engagement with feared stimuli recalibrates threat responses (Foa & Kozak, 1986),
- And **voluntary challenge**, which strengthens confidence, agency, and emotional regulation.

Within the framework of post-traumatic growth, eustress represents stress that strengthens rather than shatters. It is the physiological and psychological bridge between adversity and adaptation, activating the nervous system just enough to promote learning, resilience, and renewed capacity for meaning-making (Southwick et al., 2014; Tedeschi & Calhoun, 2018).

Forms of Controlled Discomfort Used in Recovery

Evidence-supported methods for adaptive stress exposure include:

1. Physical Challenge

Moderate resistance training, sustained postural effort (stance training such as yoga, Pilates, tai chi, martial arts, etc.), controlled endurance activity, and breath-challenging exercise increase stress tolerance, self-efficacy, and emotional stability (Ratey & Loehr, 2011; Dishman et al., 2006).

2. Thermal Stress

Brief cold exposure and controlled heat exposure improve autonomic balance, mood regulation, and stress resilience when applied conservatively (Shevchuk, 2008).

3. Emotional Exposure

Gradual engagement with avoided emotions under regulated conditions strengthens emotional tolerance and reduces avoidance-based psychopathology (Foa & Kozak, 1986).

4. Cognitive Challenge

Deliberate engagement with uncertainty, ambiguity, and complex problem-solving improves distress tolerance and cognitive flexibility (Kashdan & Rottenberg, 2010).

5. Social Stress

Healthy assertion, boundary setting, and vulnerability within safe relationships retrain interpersonal threat circuitry and attachment responses (Siegel, 2012; Porges, 2011).

Effort, Discomfort, and the Rebuilding of Agency

Trauma replaces agency with helplessness. Controlled stress rebuilds agency through voluntary effort followed by successful recovery. Each completed challenge teaches the nervous system:

- "I can tolerate discomfort."
- "I can recover."

- "I am stronger than I was."
- "Effort does not equal annihilation."

This sequence is one of the most powerful mechanisms of post-traumatic growth.
(Tedeschi & Calhoun, 2018).

The Neurochemistry of Resilience

Adaptive stress alters neurotransmitter balance in growth-supportive ways:

- Dopamine increases motivation and learning
- Norepinephrine sharpens attention
- Endorphins increase pain tolerance
- Brain-derived neurotrophic factor (BDNF) increases neuroplasticity

(Ratey & Loehr, 2011; McEwen & Wingfield, 2003).

These neurochemical changes underlie the subjective experience of resilience, confidence, and emotional stability that emerges through training.

Why Comfort Alone Does Not Produce Growth

Safety is necessary for healing, but **safety alone does not produce strength**. If recovery is limited only to comfort, the nervous system remains fragile. Growth emerges when safety and challenge are combined in balanced cycles.

Post-traumatic growth therefore requires a dialectic of rest and effort, comfort and challenge, softness and strength.

From Avoidance to Engagement

As resilience training progresses, survivors begin to shift from:

- Avoidance → Engagement
- Helplessness → Agency
- Reactivity → Choice
- Fragility → Strength
- Fear → Confidence

This shift marks a critical developmental transition in recovery: the survivor is no longer defined primarily by what overwhelms them, but by what they can now withstand.

The Role of Meaning in Stress Transformation

Stress becomes growth-producing only when it is framed by **meaning and purpose**. Without meaning, stress is merely strain. With meaning, stress becomes a forge.

Research consistently shows that meaning-making moderates the relationship between stress and psychological outcomes, transforming suffering into development when purpose is present (Park, 2010; Frankl, 2006).

Resilience as a Learned Identity

Over time, repeated cycles of effort and recovery reshape identity itself. Survivors no longer experience themselves as fragile. They experience themselves as:

- Capable
- Enduring
- Adaptive
- Grounded
- Competent under pressure

This identity shift represents one of the deepest layers of post-traumatic growth.

From Trauma Imprinting to Strength Imprinting

Trauma imprints helplessness, fear, and collapse into the nervous system. Resilience training imprints strength, endurance, and recovery. The same nervous system that once encoded terror now encodes capability. This is not symbolic. It is biological learning.

Resilience as a Cornerstone of Post-Traumatic Growth

Post-traumatic growth is not only emotional insight or cognitive reframing. It is the embodied capacity to tolerate life's pressures without fragmentation. Controlled discomfort teaches the nervous system how to stand in challenge without collapse. *When effort no longer equals threat, the survivor becomes free to engage life fully. This is the rebirth of resilience.*

Rewiring the Human Nervous System: Adapting to a High-Voltage World

The human nervous system can be likened to an electrical system designed for specific voltage and amperage. Traditionally, it is assumed that most individuals are wired for 110 volts and 10 amps. However, contemporary society necessitates functioning at 220 volts and 30 amps, far exceeding the capacity originally intended by our biology. This increased "voltage" manifests as chronic stress, anxiety, burnout, and various physical ailments.

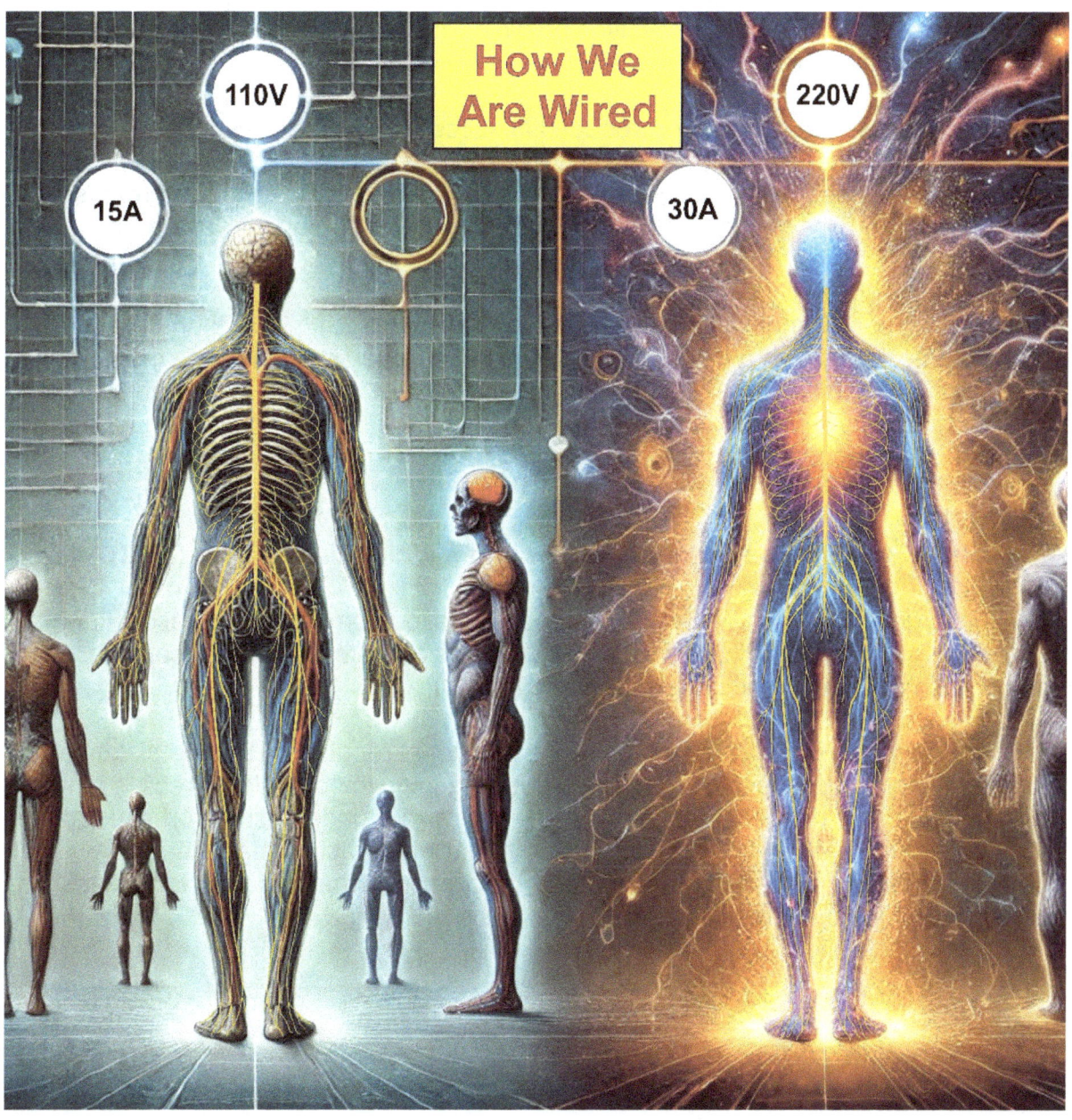

Nevertheless, just as an electrical system can be rewired to handle greater loads, the human nervous system can also be trained to adapt. Ancient practices such as martial arts, qigong, Dao Yin (Taoist yoga), yoga, and breathwork serve as effective interventions. These time-tested methods bridge the gap between the body's inherent capabilities and the demands of modern life, enabling the nervous system to withstand higher levels of stress without succumbing to being overwhelmed.

The Role of Stance Training and Controlled Stress

With over 45 years of experience in martial arts, qigong, Dao Yin, and yoga, I have observed that certain methods can effectively enhance the nervous system. One such method is stance training, which involves holding postures for specific durations while integrating breath control.

For beginners, basic stances are introduced in succession, initially without prolonged holds. As they progress, duration gradually increases. Once students can hold each stance for 30 seconds, controlled breathing is incorporated, typically three breaths per 30 seconds. With consistent practice, the duration is extended to one-minute holds, adjusting breath cycles to around four to six respirations per minute.

This approach serves multiple purposes. On a physical level, it strengthens the legs, core, and other stabilizing muscles. On a neurological level, it encourages the nervous system to adapt to discomfort, fostering resilience, endurance, and focus. On an energetic level, it stimulates the body's internal pathways, potentially leading to enhanced vitality and internal balance.

The Science Behind the Training: The Anterior Midcingulate Cortex (aMCC)

While these practices have been in use for centuries, contemporary neuroscience provides insight into their effectiveness. A critical region of the brain implicated in resilience is the anterior midcingulate cortex (aMCC).

The aMCC is responsible for effortful control, emotional regulation, and persistence in the face of challenges. Research indicates that engaging in controlled stress, such as maintaining difficult stances, regulating breath, or training under discomfort strengthens and enlarging the aMCC. Consequently, individuals who practice these methods may enhance their ability to manage stress more effectively, increase mental toughness, and maintain composure under pressure.

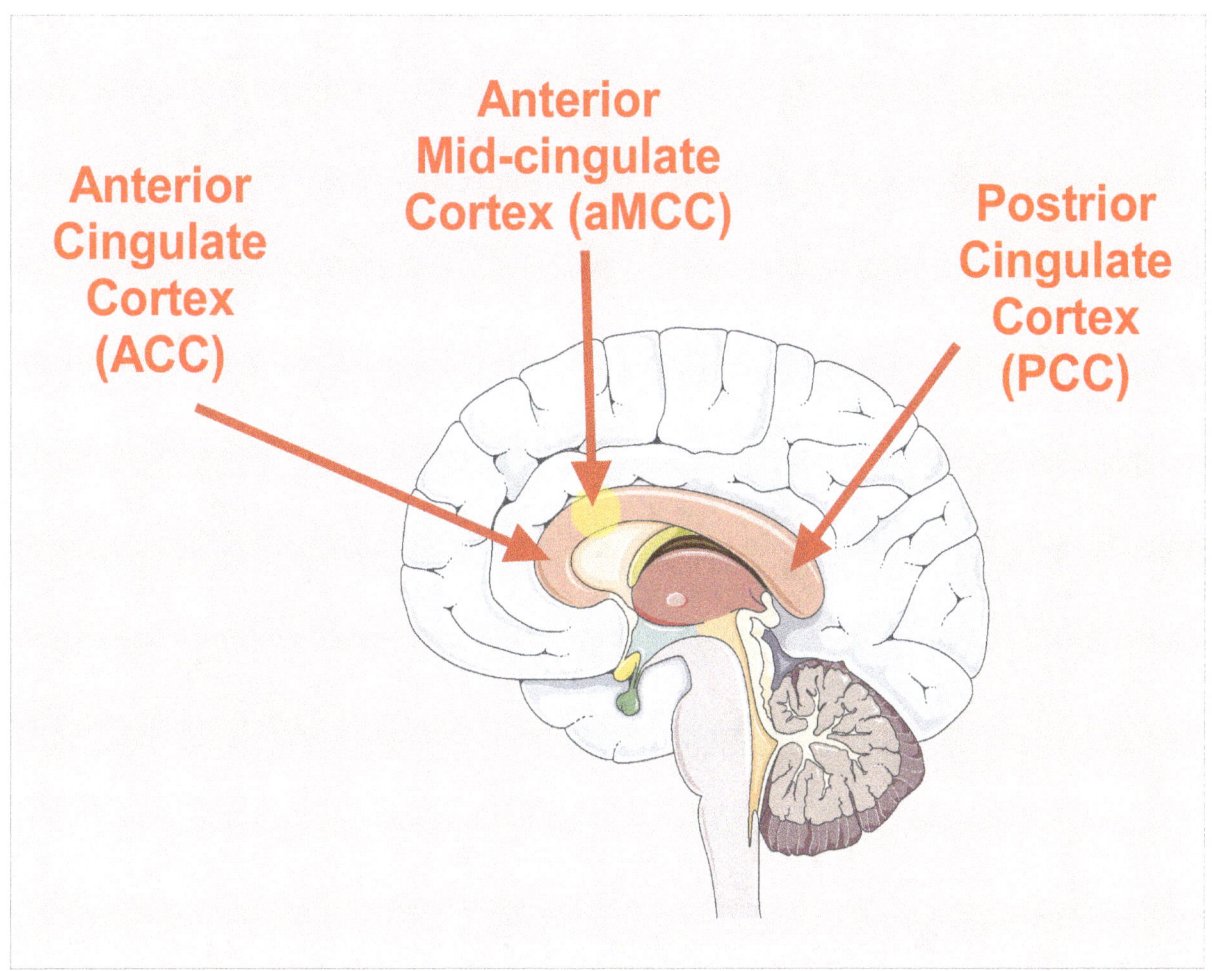

In essence, deliberate training can augment our capacity to handle life's challenges, analogous to how lifting heavier weights strengthens muscles. This concept is consistent with the principle of progressive overload, which is well-established in strength training and equally applicable to the nervous system and mental resilience.

"Burning the *Chong Mai"* – The Energetic Dimension

Beyond the physical and neurological aspects, these practices have deep roots in Taoist and Traditional Chinese Medicine (TCM). An important concept in energetic cultivation is "burning the Chong Mai."

The Chong Mai (Thrusting Vessel) is one of the eight extraordinary meridians in TCM. It serves as a primary channel for deep energy reserves, influencing the body's overall energy flow. When stance work and controlled breathing are practiced regularly, this meridian can be activated, which may allow for greater energy circulation through the other seven extraordinary vessels and the twelve main meridians.

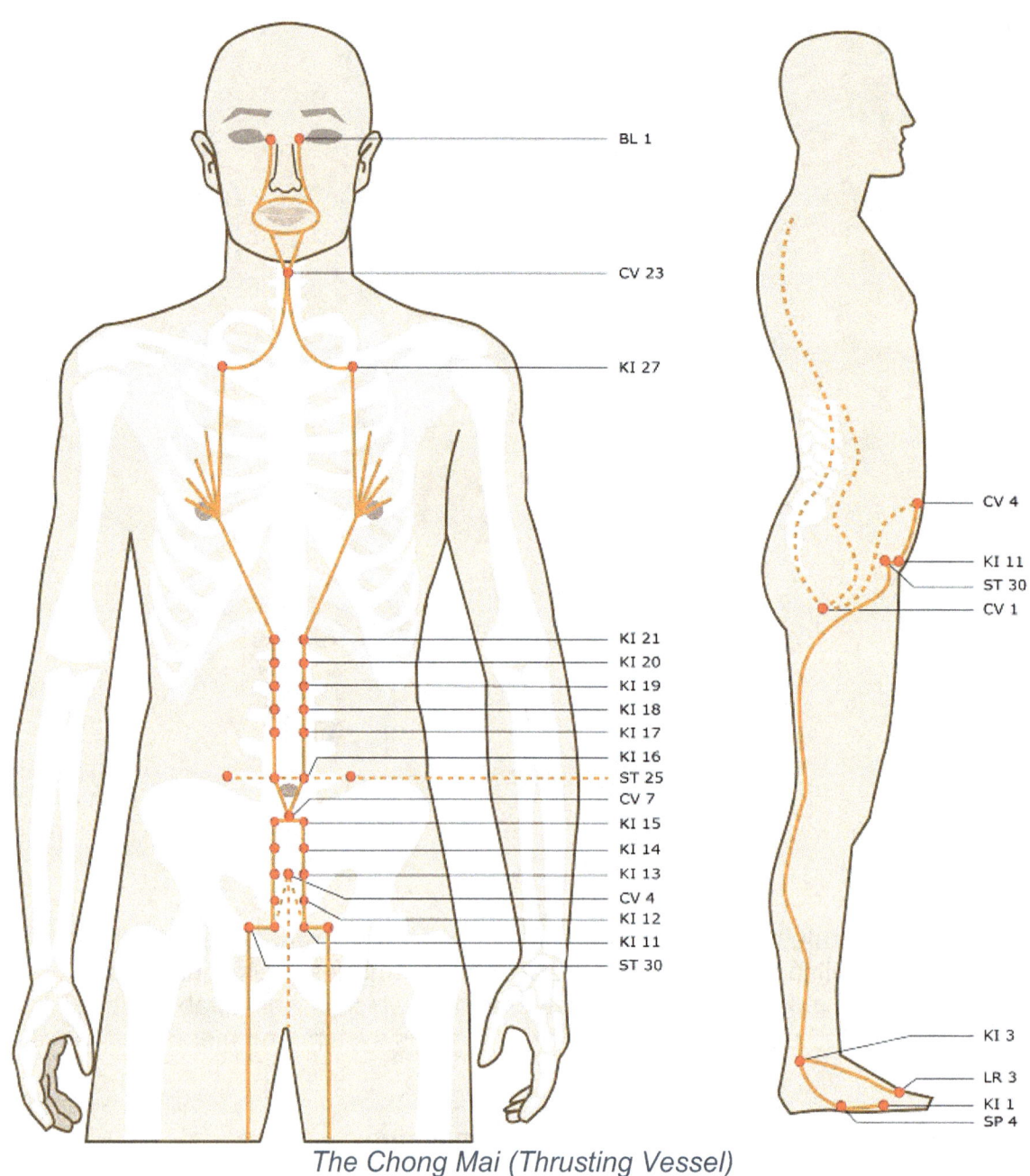

The Chong Mai (Thrusting Vessel)

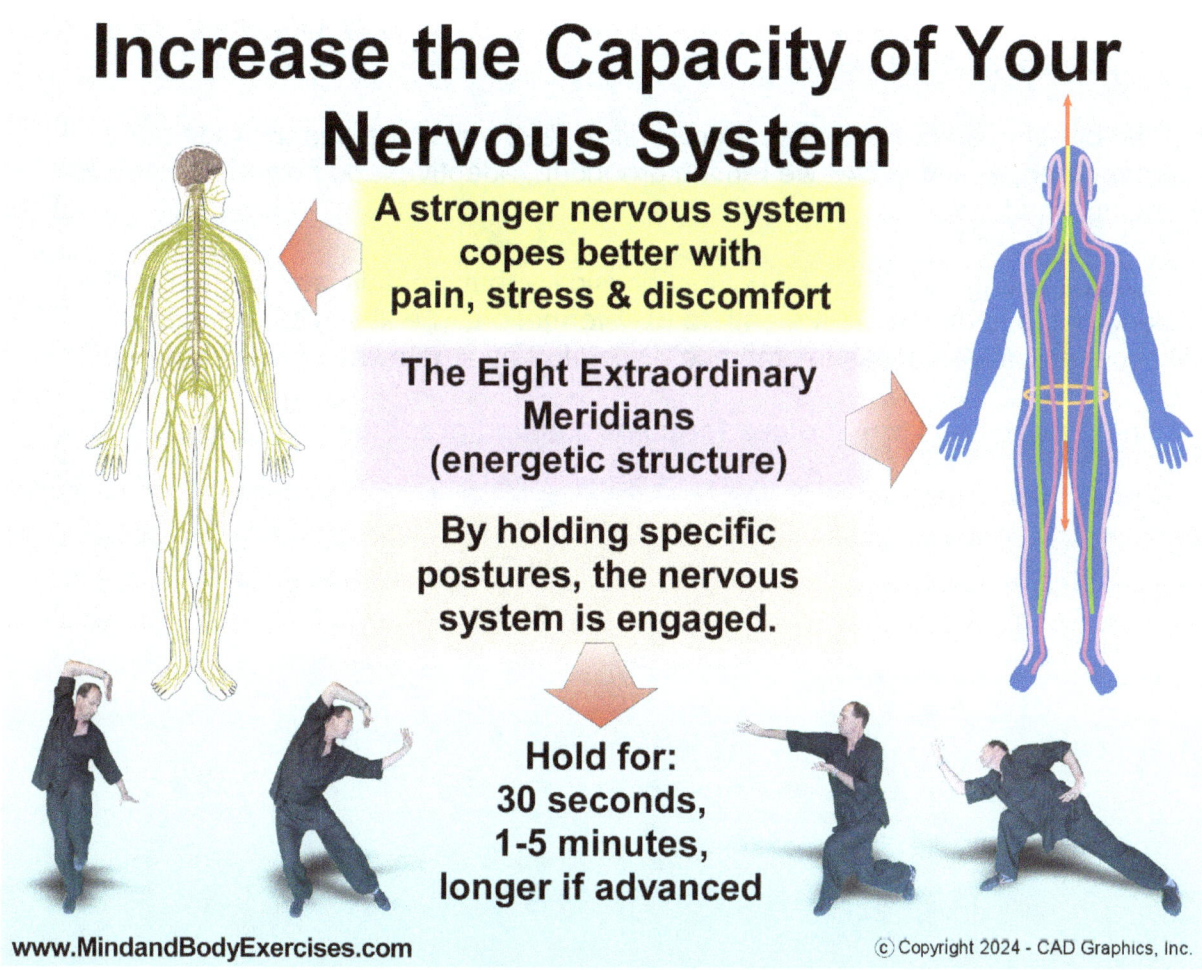

This process can be compared to upgrading a power grid. By increasing the capacity of the Chong Mai, the entire energetic system can become more efficient, stable, and resilient. This observation might explain why long-term practitioners of qigong, Dao Yin, and martial arts often report higher energy levels, improved focus, and a significant sense of internal strength.

Resilience Through Discomfort: The Path to Transformation

The old adage *"That which does not kill us makes us stronger"* perfectly encapsulates the philosophy behind these training methods. Rather than avoiding stress, we use it as a tool for growth.

- **Physically**, stance training builds strength, endurance, and structural integrity.
- **Mentally**, breath control and effortful posture-holding train the nervous system to remain calm under pressure.
- **Neurologically**, the aMCC adapts and strengthens, improving stress management and persistence.

- **Energetically**, activating the Chong Mai and meridian system enhances internal power and resilience.

Instead of being overwhelmed by modern life's "220 volts," we can upgrade our own internal wiring, ensuring that we remain grounded, adaptive, and powerful in an ever-changing world.

For those seeking true strength, not just physically, but mentally and spiritually, these ancient methods offer a proven path to transformation. The key is consistency, patience, and a willingness to embrace discomfort as a gateway to resilience.

(see next pages and appendices for color detailed graphics on these practices)

Filling the 8 Vessels

www.MindAndBodyExercises.com

8 Vessels

The 8 Extraordinary Vessels are part of the body's meridian energy system. These vessels serve as reservoirs for the 12 Regular meridians. Above all else, they regulate the excess and lack of energy within the other meridians, These vessels are located in close proximity to the other meridians, often-times intersecting or running parallel with them.

12 Meridians
Lung
Heart
Pericardium
Large Intestine
Small Intestine
Triple Burner
Spleen
Kidney
Liver
Heart
Stomach
Bladder
Gall Bladder

8 Vessels
Conception
Governing
Thrusting
Belt
Yin Linking
Yang Linking
Yin Heel
Yang Heel

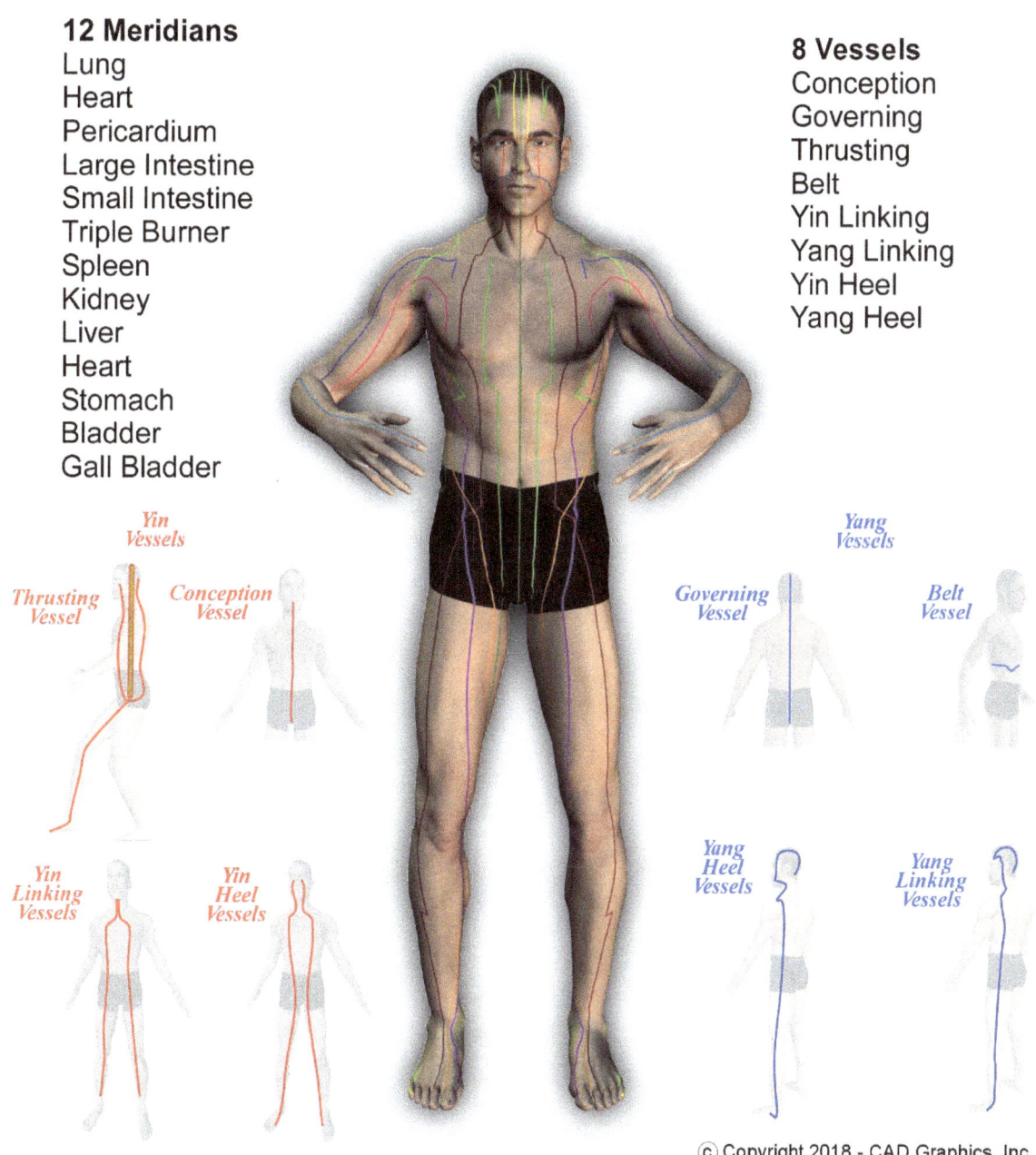

© Copyright 2018 - CAD Graphics, Inc.

61

The Eight Extraordinary Meridians

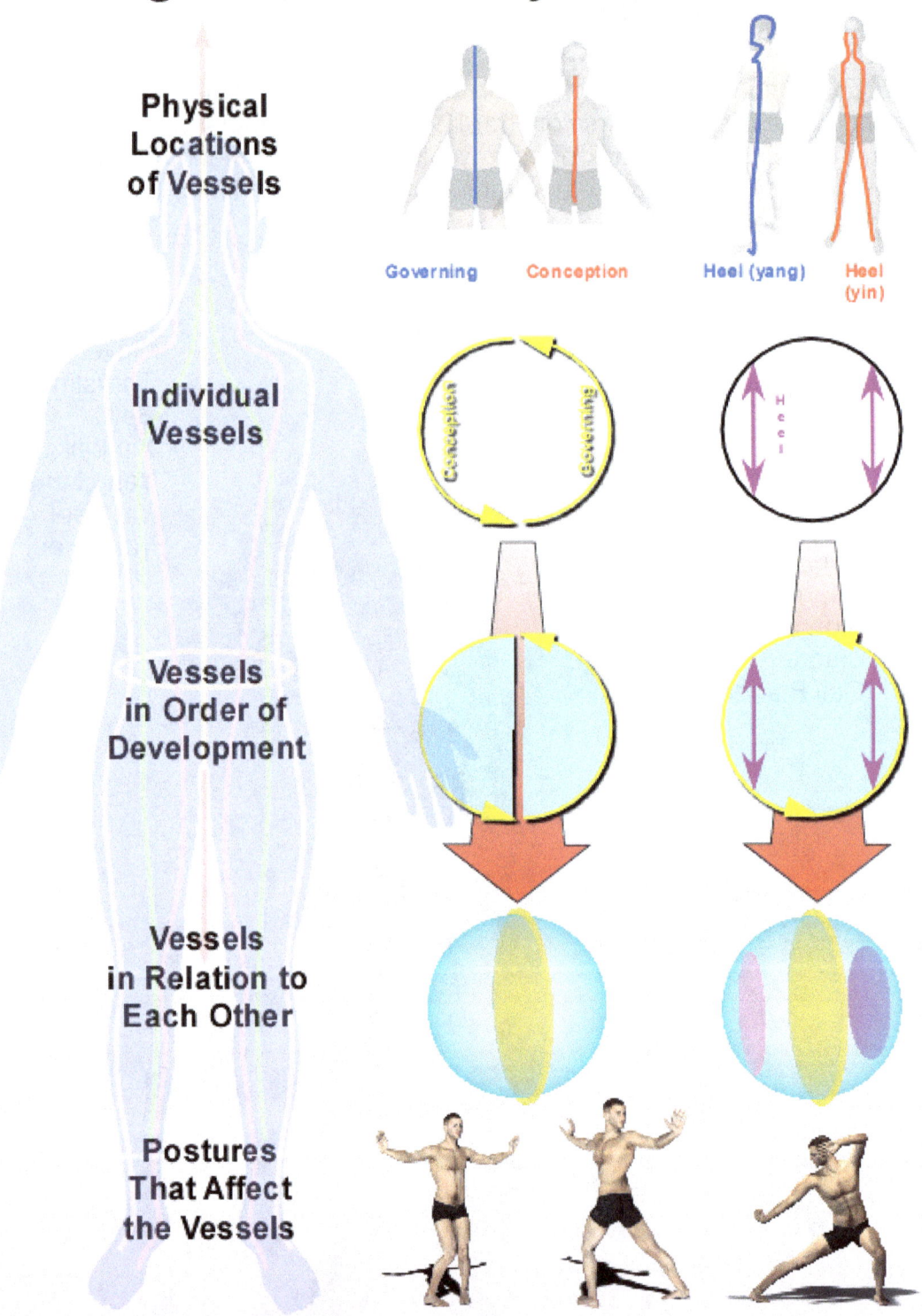

www.MindAndBodyExercises.com

(energetic structure)

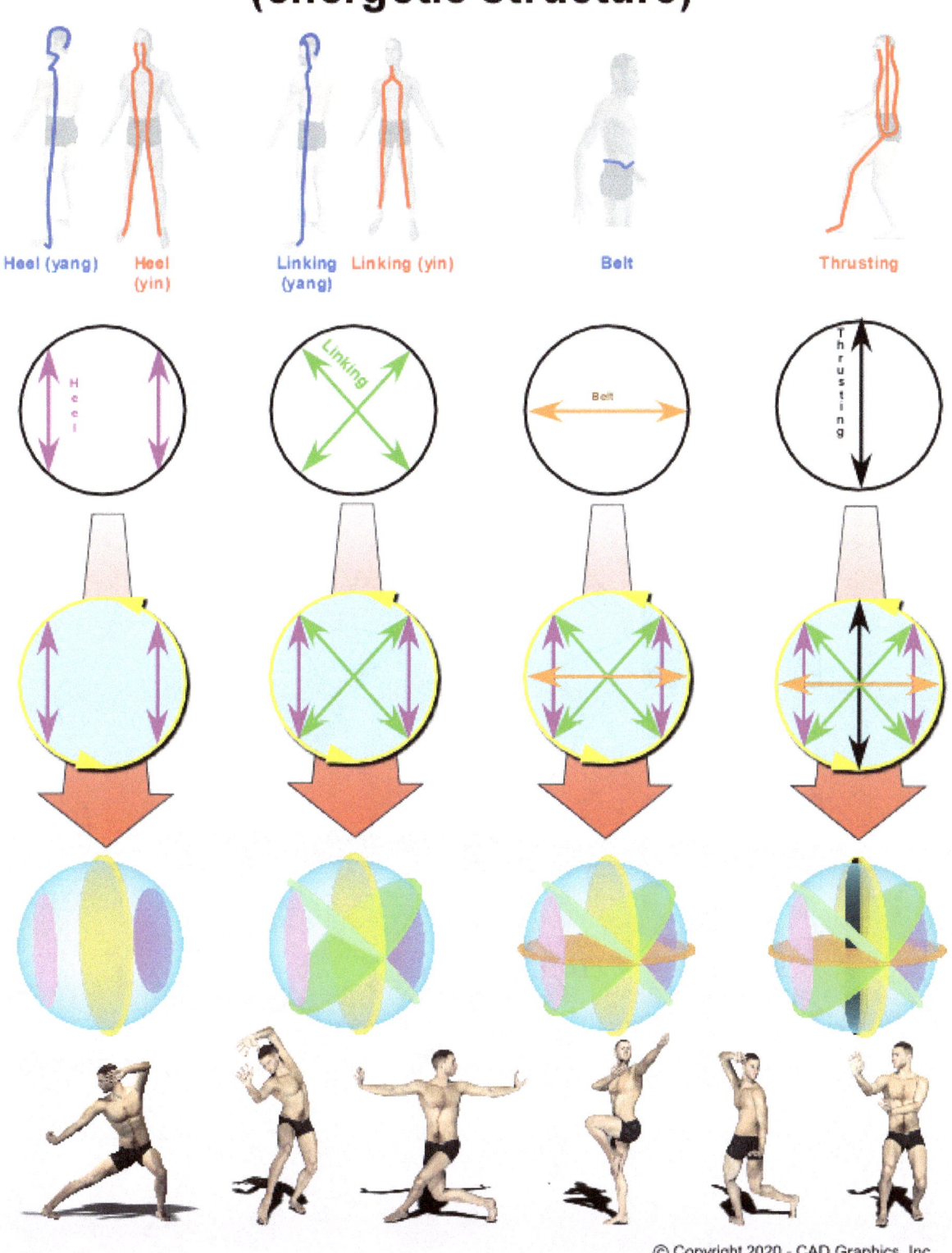

Introductory Set

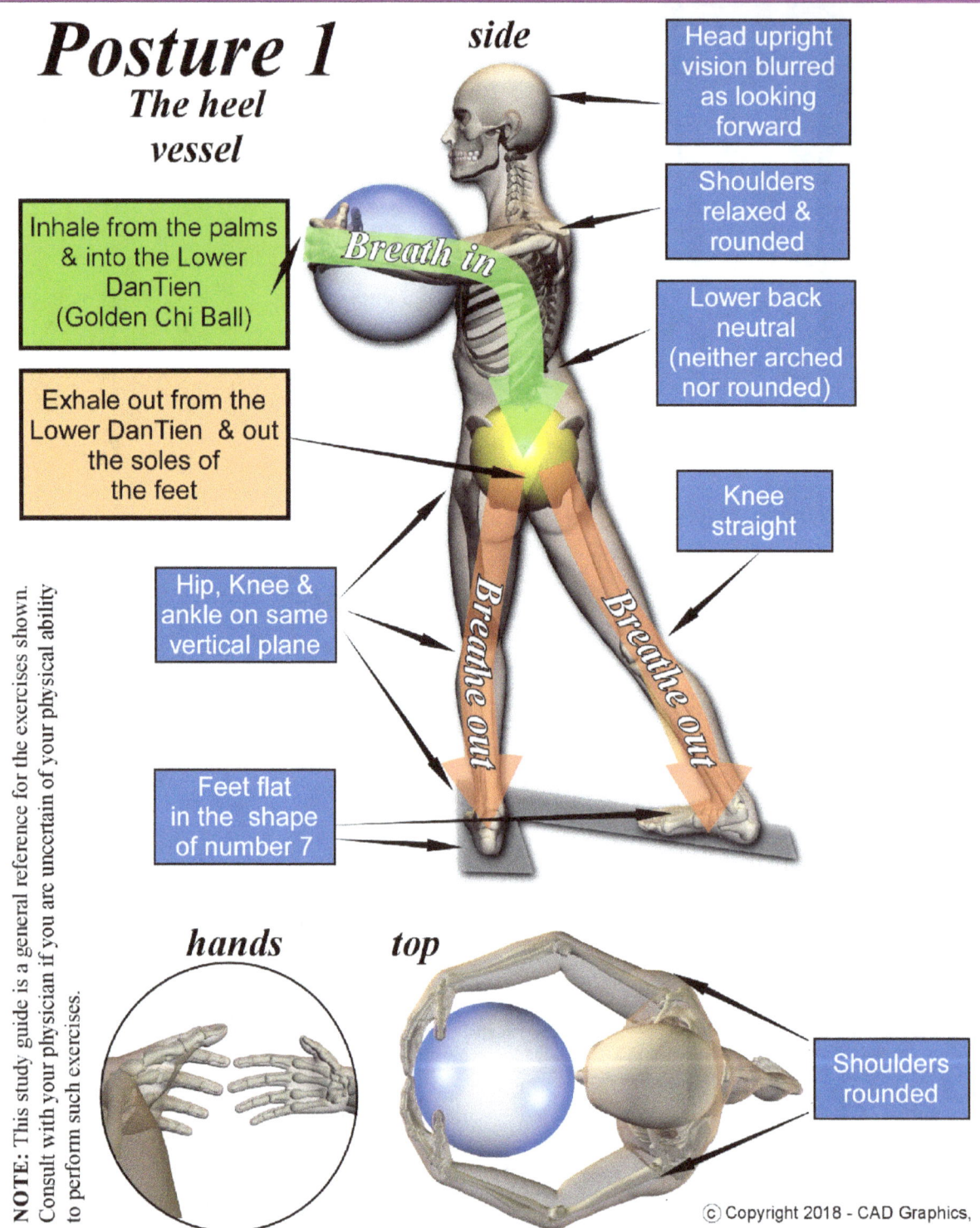

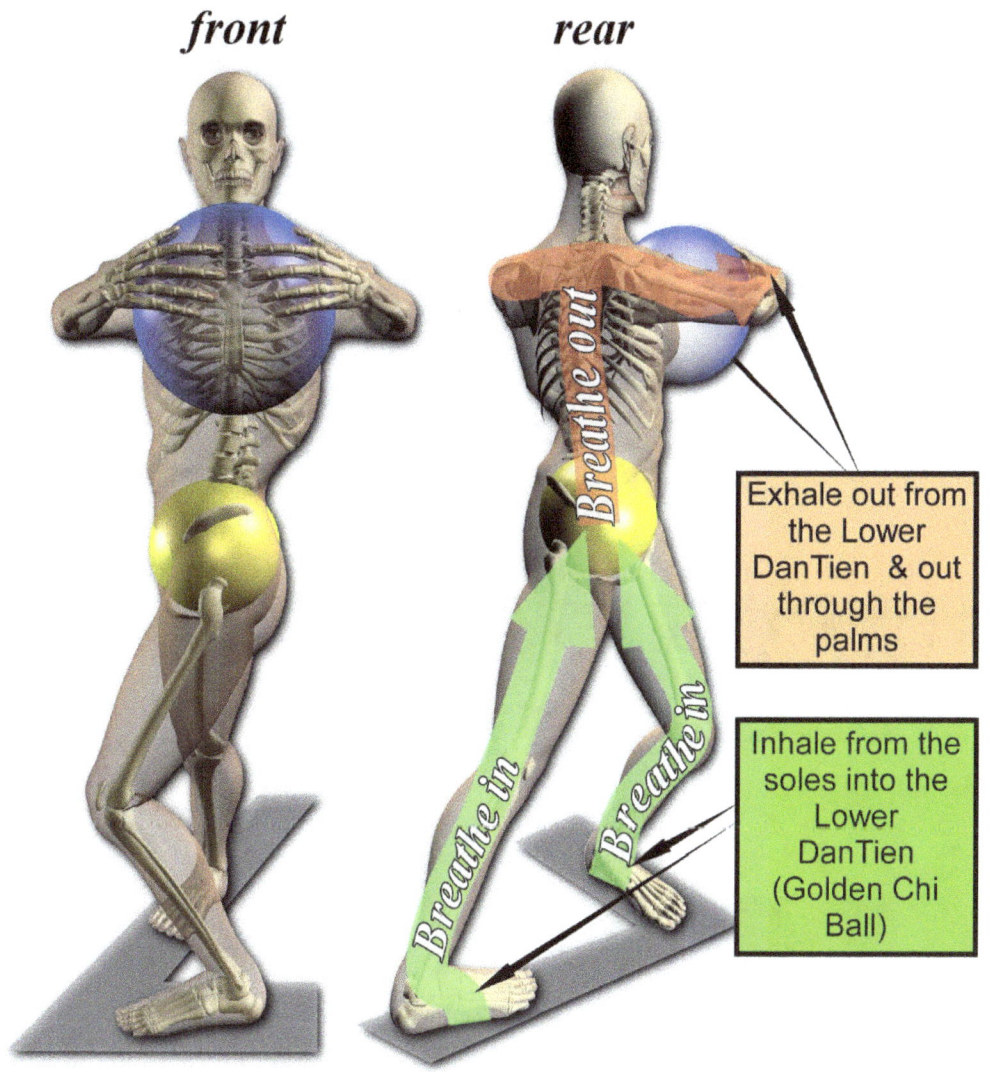

Set 1 activates all 9 gates as well as preparing the muscles, joints and bones for the next progressive stances. Start with the feet, working your way up the body as applying the proper positions and posture. Imagine holding a weightless ball between your palms and chest for this 1st exercise. Inhale from palms down into the Lower DanTien. Exhale from this point and out through the soles of the feet. Inhale from the soles into the DanTien. Exhale out from the DanTien and through to the palms to complete 1 full repetition. Execute on both sides for 1 set.

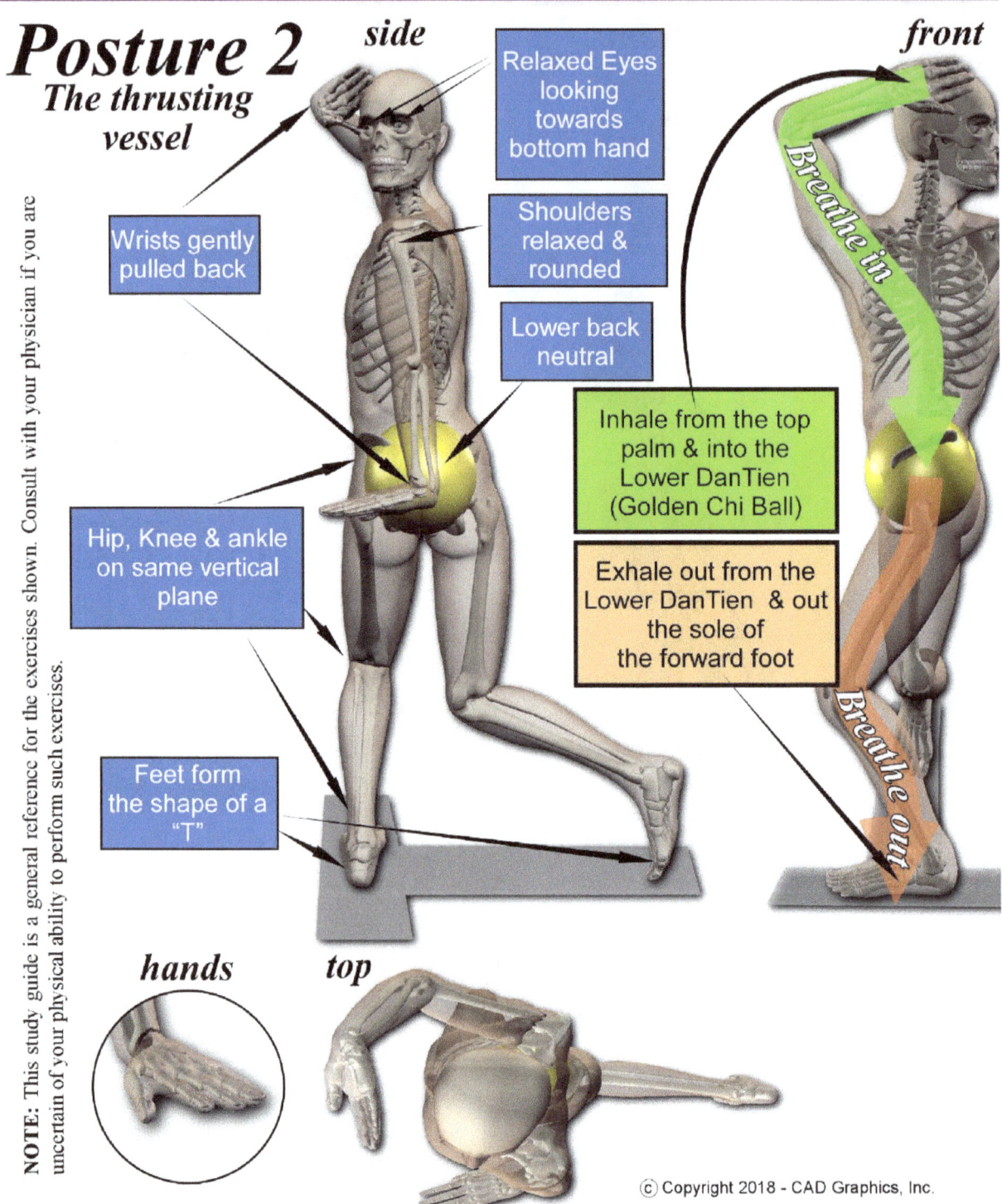

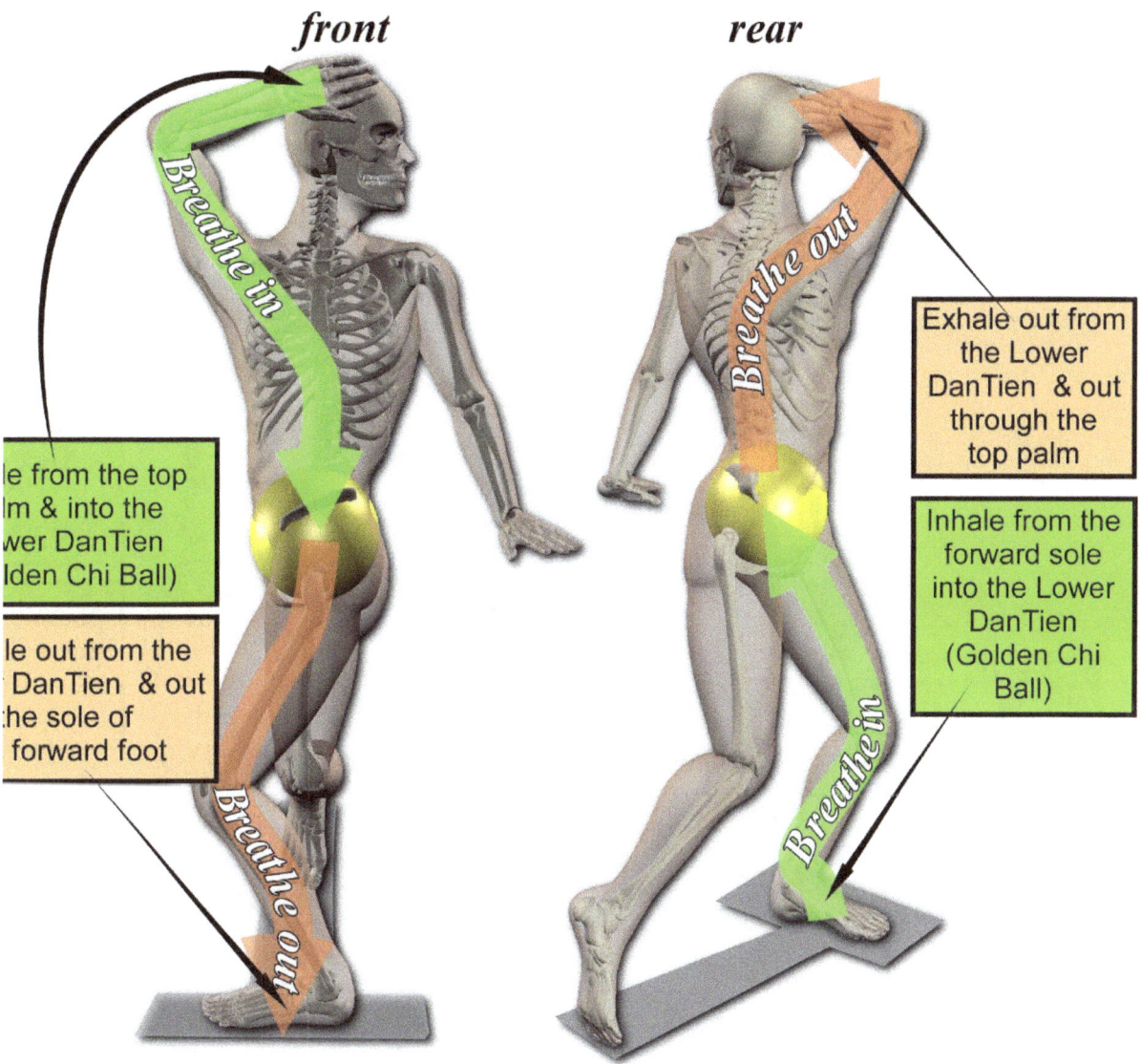

Set 2 also activates all 9 gates while putting extra resistance on the hips, thighs and ankles. Start with the feet, working your way up the body as applying the proper positions and posture. Inhale from upward palm down into the Lower DanTien. Exhale from this point and out through the sole of the forward foot. Inhale from the sole into the DanTien. Exhale out from the DanTien and through the palm to complete 1 full repetition. Execute on both sides for 1 set.

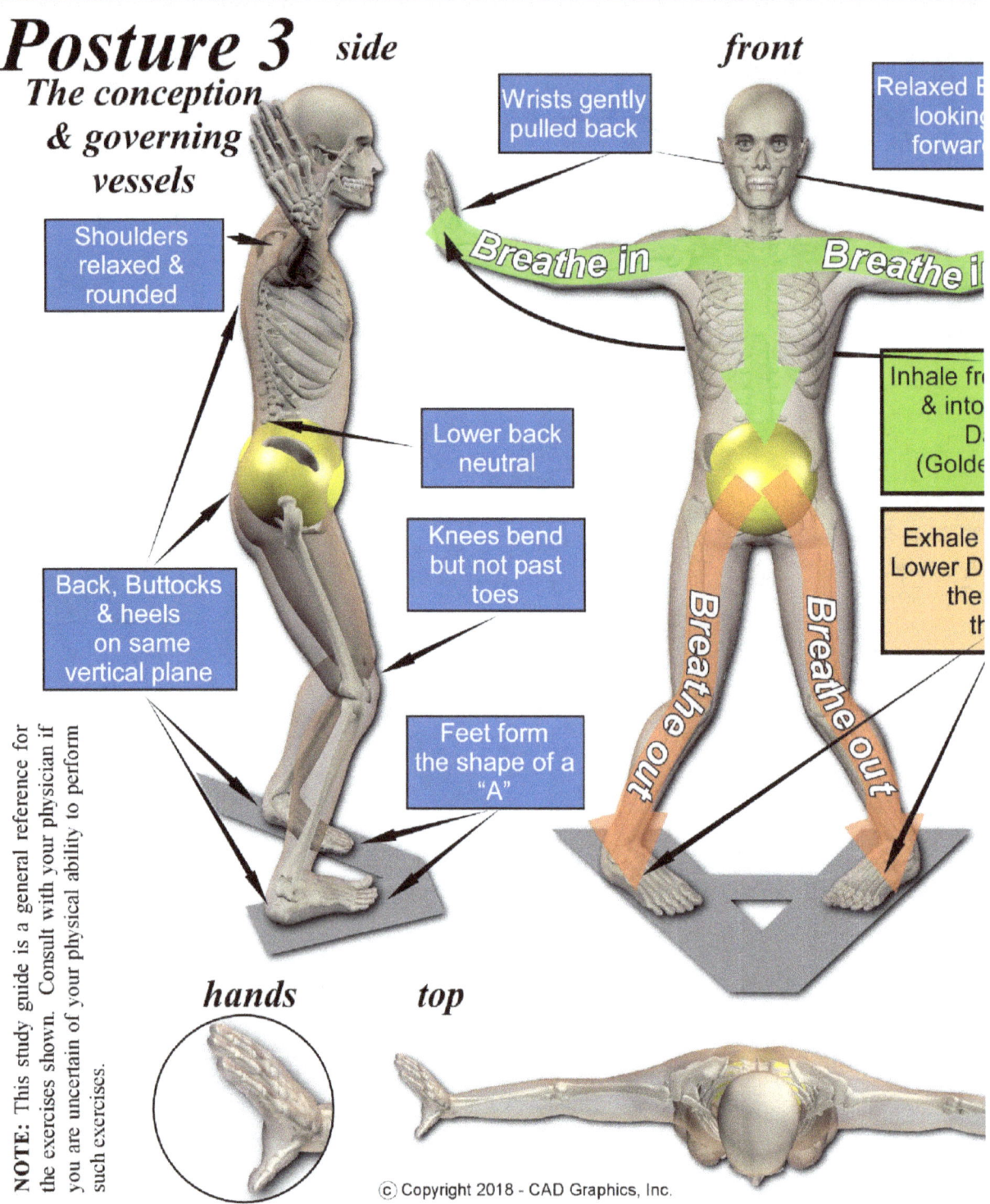

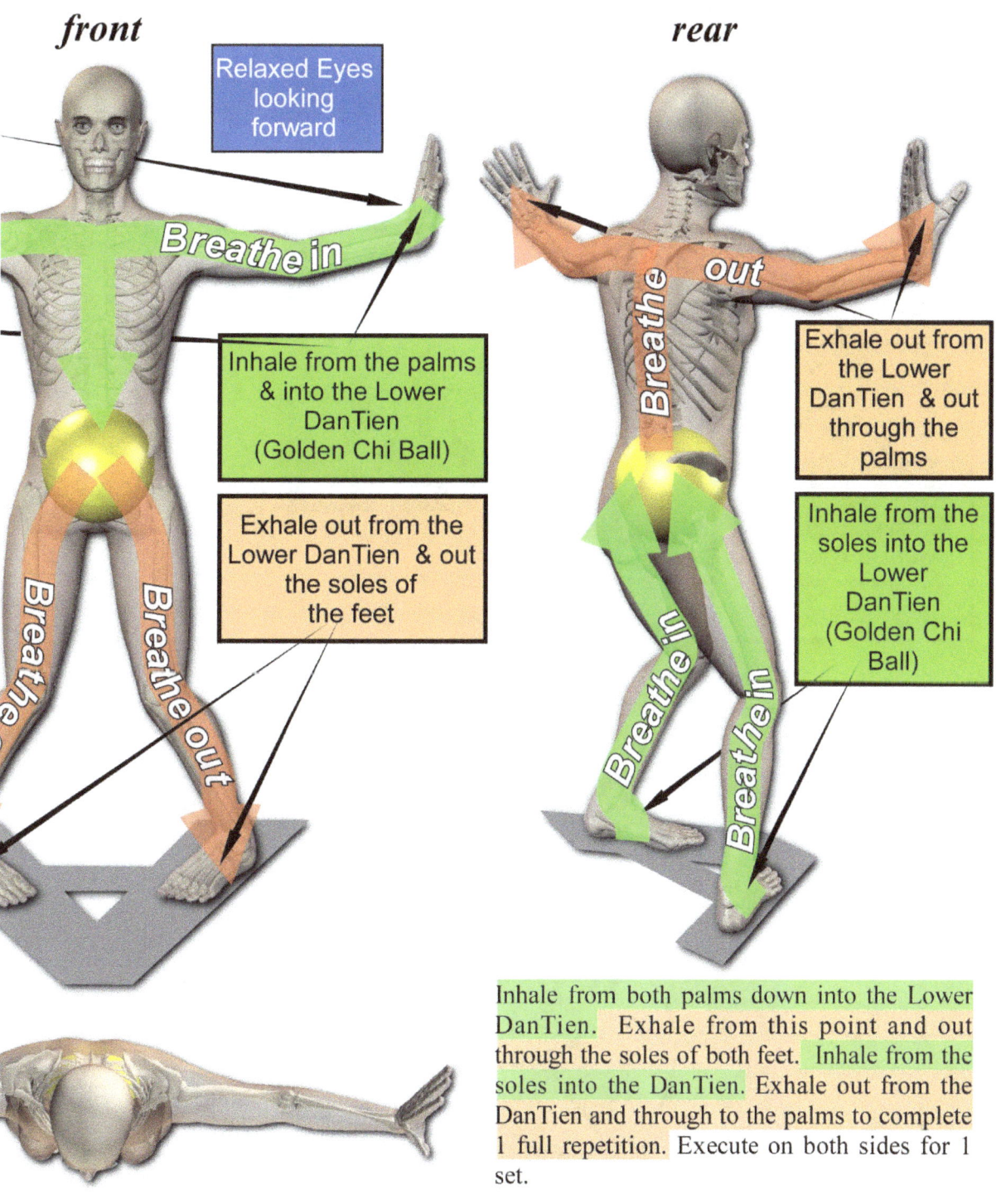

Inhale from both palms down into the Lower DanTien. Exhale from this point and out through the soles of both feet. Inhale from the soles into the DanTien. Exhale out from the DanTien and through to the palms to complete 1 full repetition. Execute on both sides for 1 set.

Introductory Set

Posture 4
The belt vessel

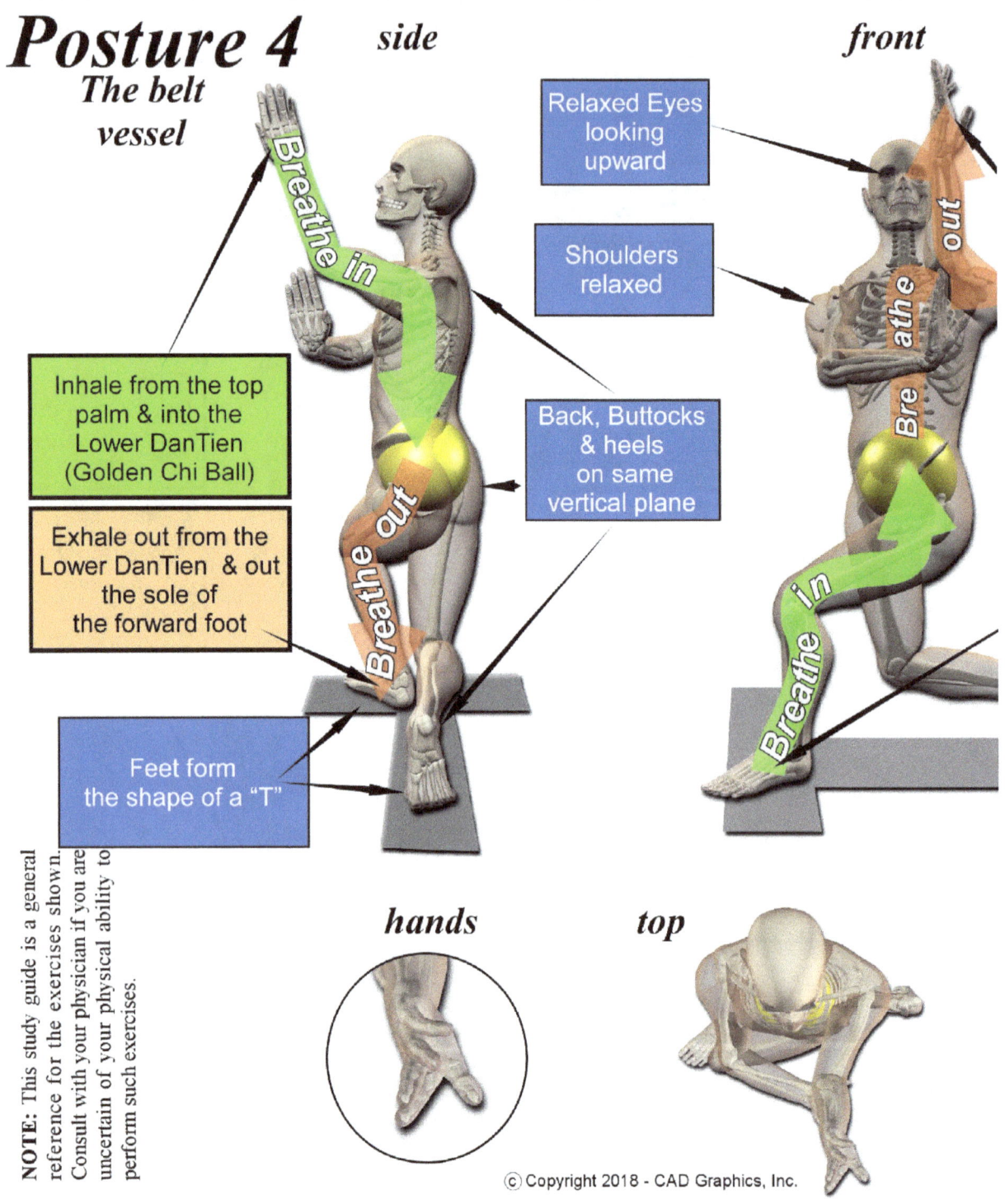

- Inhale from the top palm & into the Lower DanTien (Golden Chi Ball)
- Exhale out from the Lower DanTien & out the sole of the forward foot
- Relaxed Eyes looking upward
- Shoulders relaxed
- Back, Buttocks & heels on same vertical plane
- Feet form the shape of a "T"

side / *front* / *hands* / *top*

NOTE: This study guide is a general reference for the exercises shown. Consult with your physician if you are uncertain of your physical ability to perform such exercises.

© Copyright 2018 - CAD Graphics, Inc.

www.MindAndBodyExercises.com

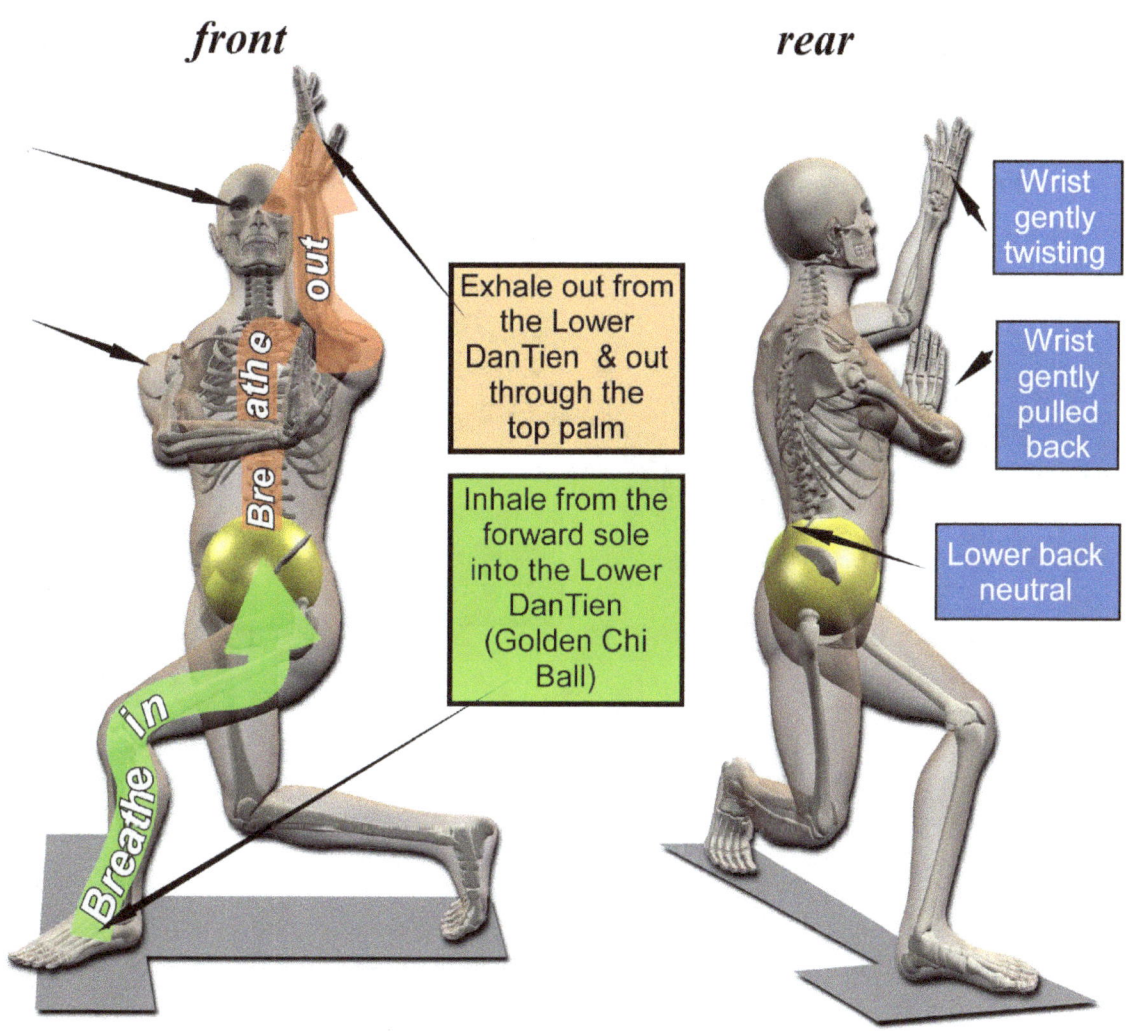

Set 4 stimulates the belt vessel by twisting the torso like a wet dish towel. This stance also strengthens the thighs, knees and ankles. Start with the feet, working your way up the body as applying the proper positions and posture. Inhale from upward palm down into the Lower DanTien. Exhale from this point and out through the sole of the forward foot. Inhale from the sole into the DanTien. Exhale out from the DanTien and through the palm to complete 1 full repetition. Execute on both sides for 1 set.

Introductory Set

Posture 5
The linking vessel

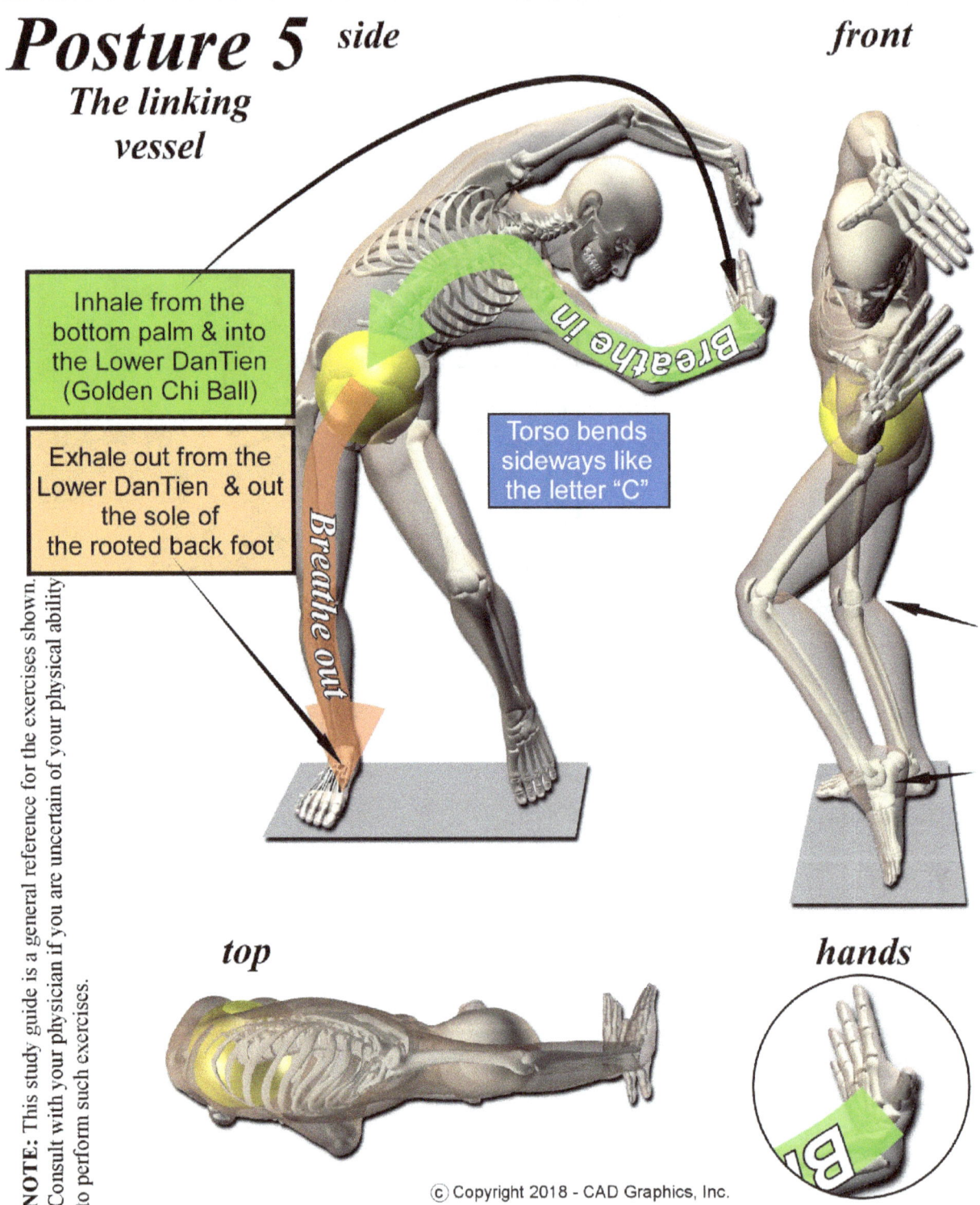

side *front*

Inhale from the bottom palm & into the Lower DanTien (Golden Chi Ball)

Exhale out from the Lower DanTien & out the sole of the rooted back foot

Torso bends sideways like the letter "C"

top *hands*

NOTE: This study guide is a general reference for the exercises shown. Consult with your physician if you are uncertain of your physical ability to perform such exercises.

© Copyright 2018 - CAD Graphics, Inc.

72

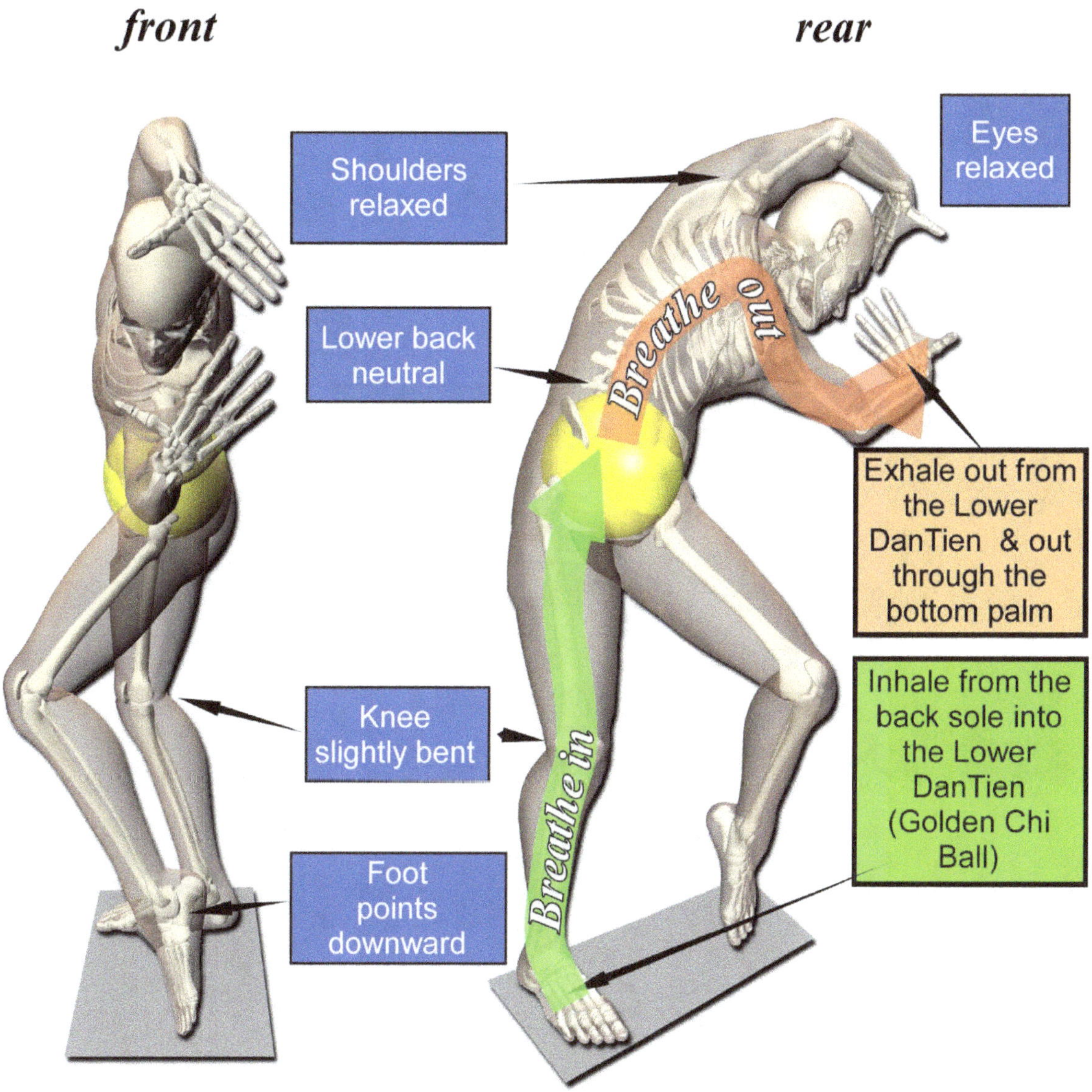

www.MindAndBodyExercises.com

front   *rear*

- Shoulders relaxed
- Eyes relaxed
- Lower back neutral
- Exhale out from the Lower DanTien & out through the bottom palm
- Inhale from the back sole into the Lower DanTien (Golden Chi Ball)
- Knee slightly bent
- Foot points downward

Breathe out / Breathe in

hands

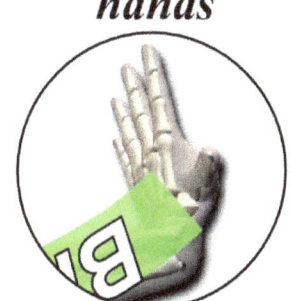

Set 5 increases the range of motion in the spine and torso. Start with the feet, working your way up the body as applying the proper positions and posture. Inhale from bottom palm down into the Lower DanTien. Exhale from this point and out through the sole of the rooted back foot. Inhale from the sole into the DanTien. Exhale out from the DanTien and through the palm to complete 1 full repetition. Execute on both sides for 1 set.

Introductory Set

Posture 6
The thrusting vessel

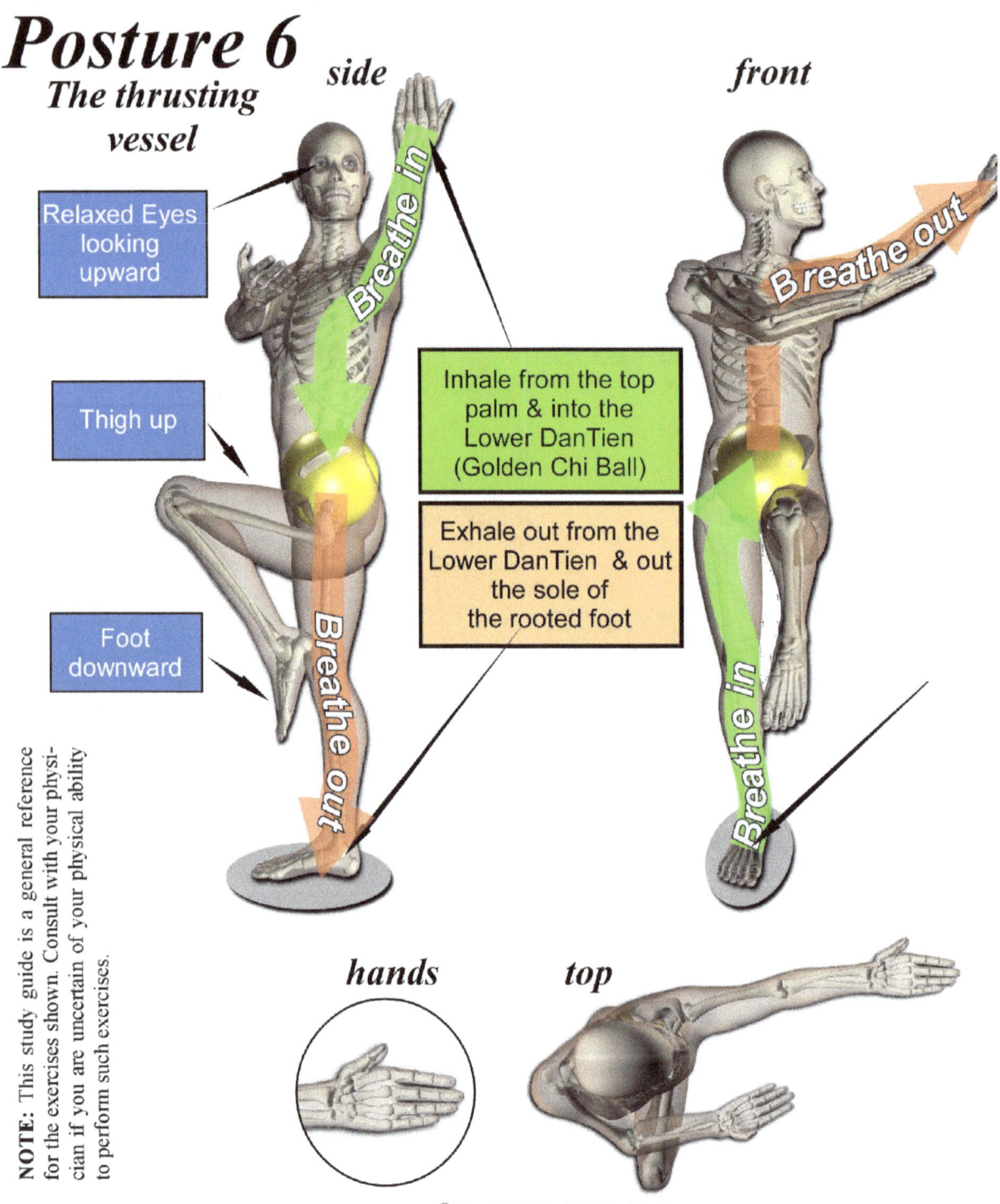

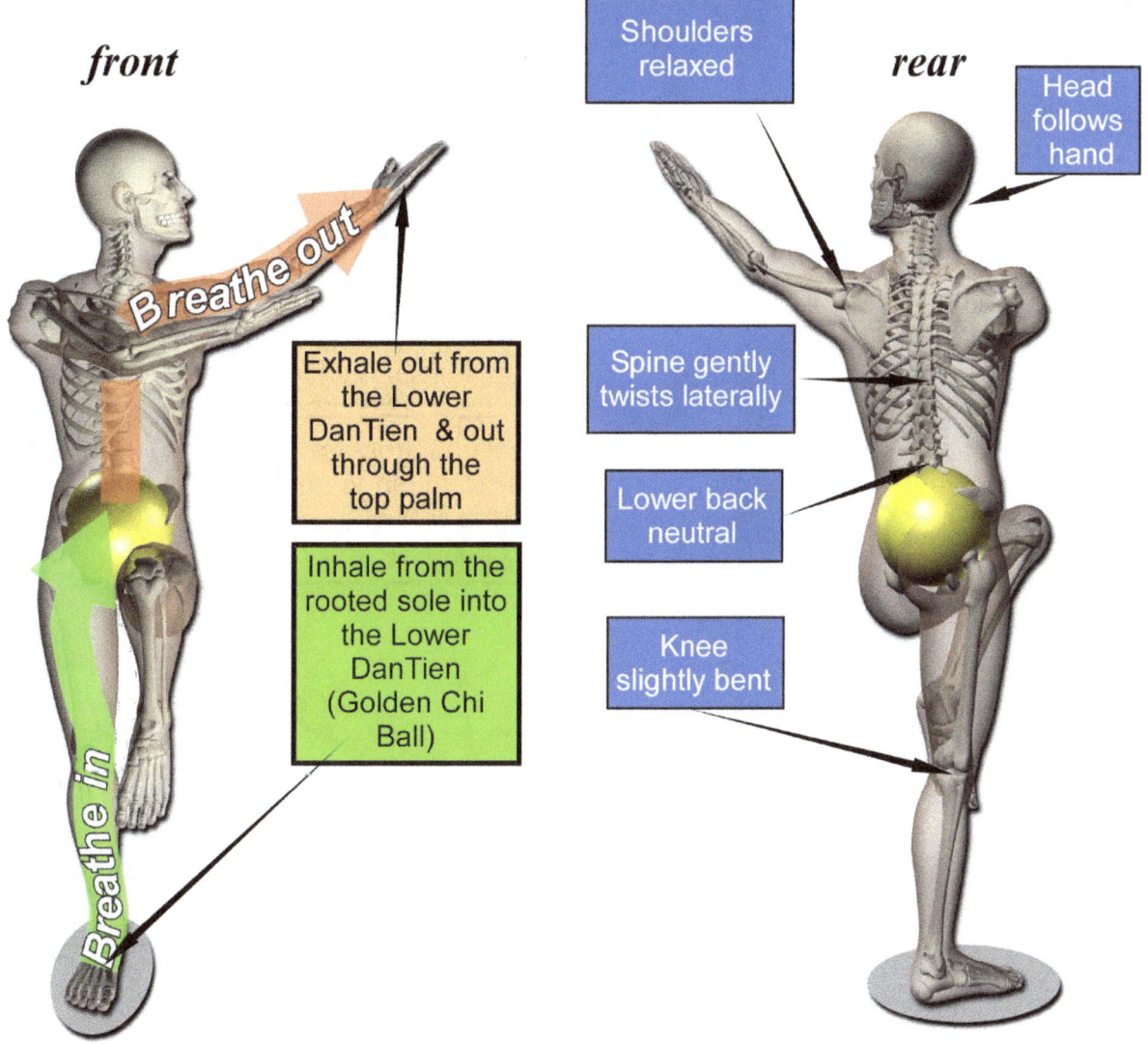

Set 6 increases balance and focus. Start with the feet, working your way up the body as applying the proper positions and posture. Inhale from upward palm down into the Lower DanTien. Exhale from this point and out through the sole of the rooted foot. Inhale from the sole into the DanTien. Exhale out from the DanTien and through the palm to complete 1 full repetition. Execute on both sides for 1 set.

Introductory Set

Posture 7 — *side*
The heel vessel

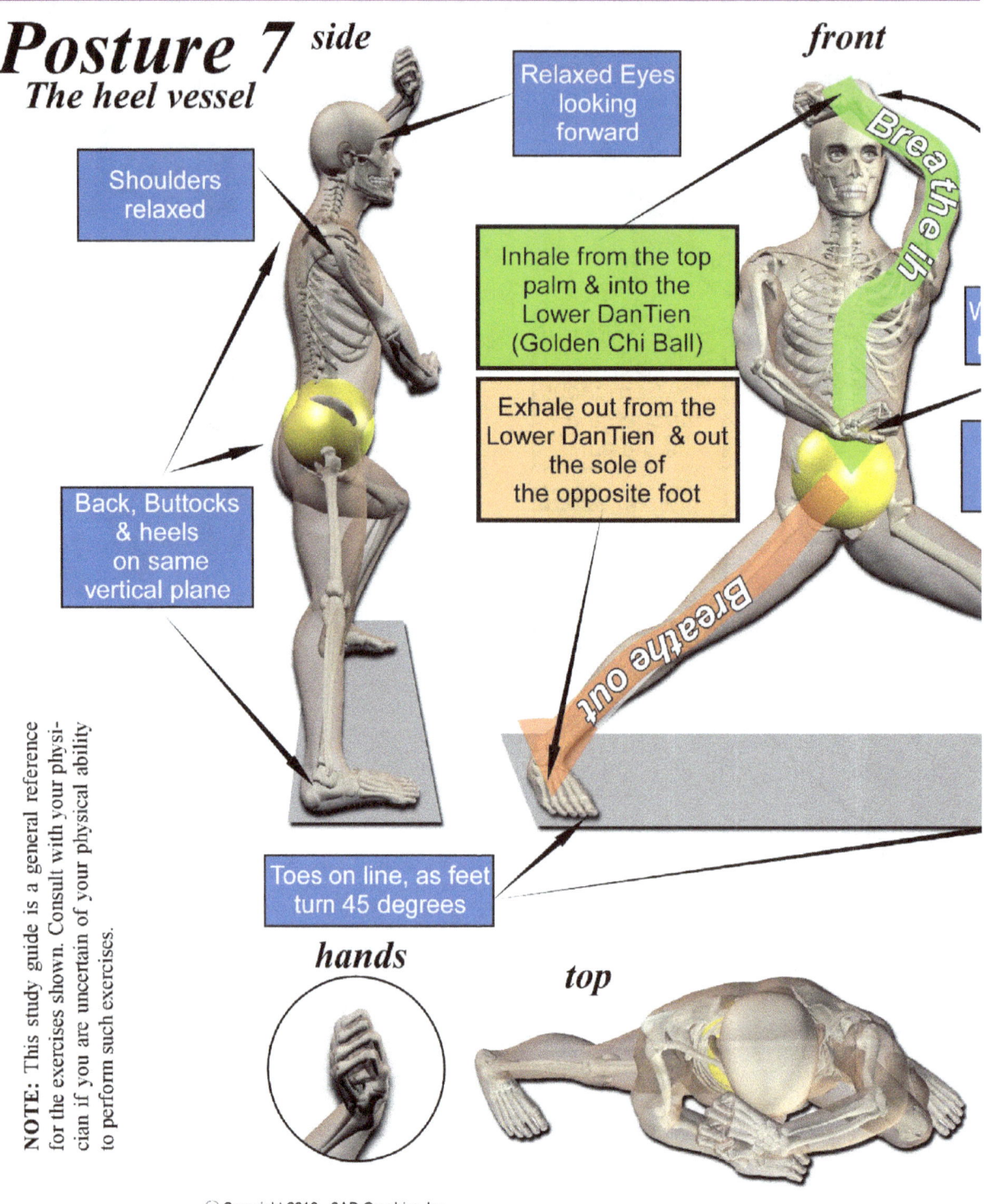

- Relaxed Eyes looking forward
- Shoulders relaxed
- Inhale from the top palm & into the Lower DanTien (Golden Chi Ball)
- Exhale out from the Lower DanTien & out the sole of the opposite foot
- Back, Buttocks & heels on same vertical plane
- Toes on line, as feet turn 45 degrees
- Breathe in / Breathe out

front · *hands* · *top*

NOTE: This study guide is a general reference for the exercises shown. Consult with your physician if you are uncertain of your physical ability to perform such exercises.

© Copyright 2018 - CAD Graphics, Inc.

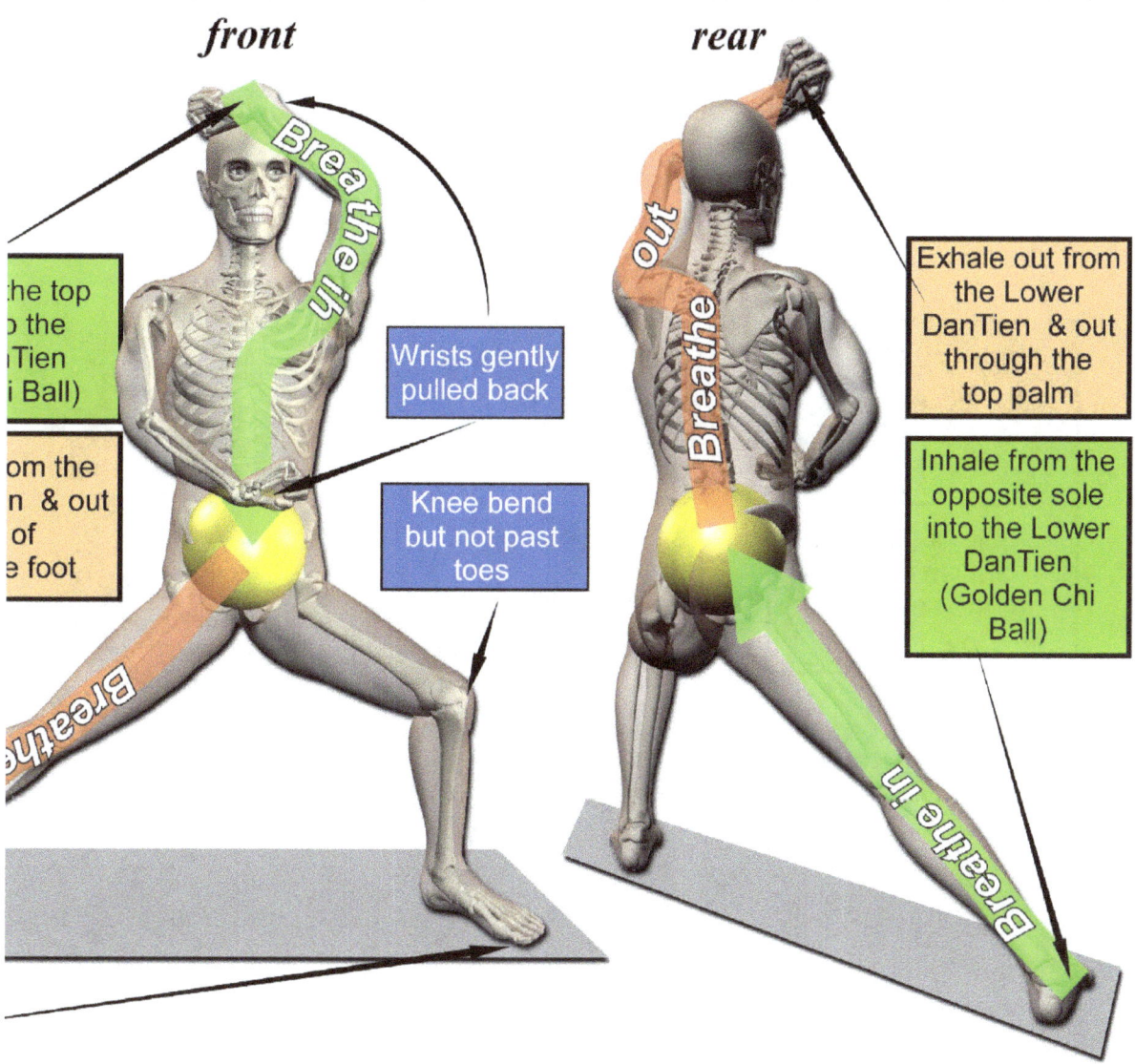

Set 7 strengthens and stretches muscles within the hips, thighs and lower back. Start with the feet, working your way up the body as applying the proper positions and posture. Inhale from upward palm down into the Lower DanTien. Exhale from this point and out through the sole of the opposite foot. Inhale from the sole into the DanTien. Exhale out from the DanTien and through the palm to complete 1 full repetition. Execute on both sides for 1 set.

Introductory Set

Posture 8
The thrusting vessel

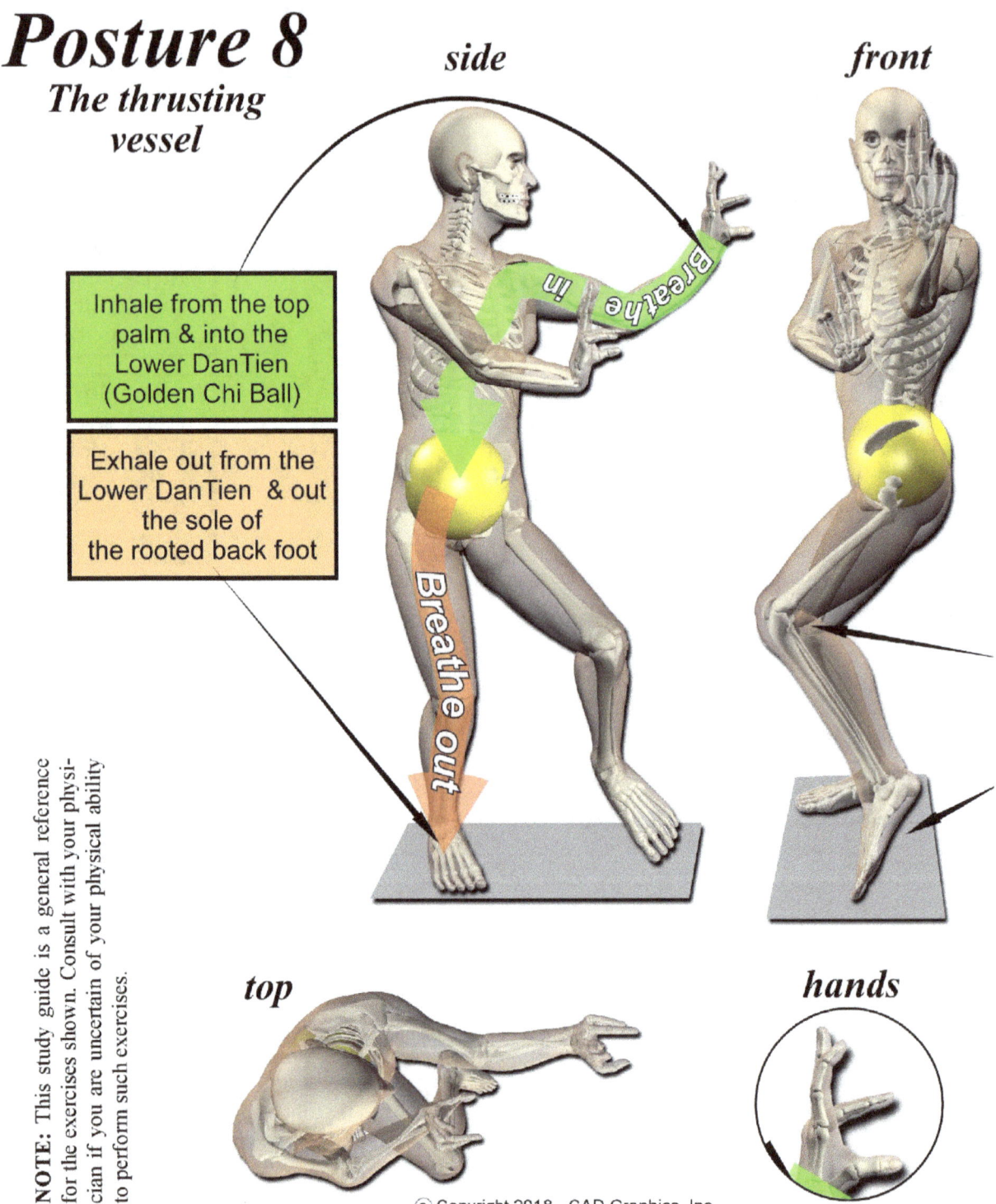

Inhale from the top palm & into the Lower DanTien (Golden Chi Ball)

Exhale out from the Lower DanTien & out the sole of the rooted back foot

NOTE: This study guide is a general reference for the exercises shown. Consult with your physician if you are uncertain of your physical ability to perform such exercises.

© Copyright 2018 - CAD Graphics, Inc.

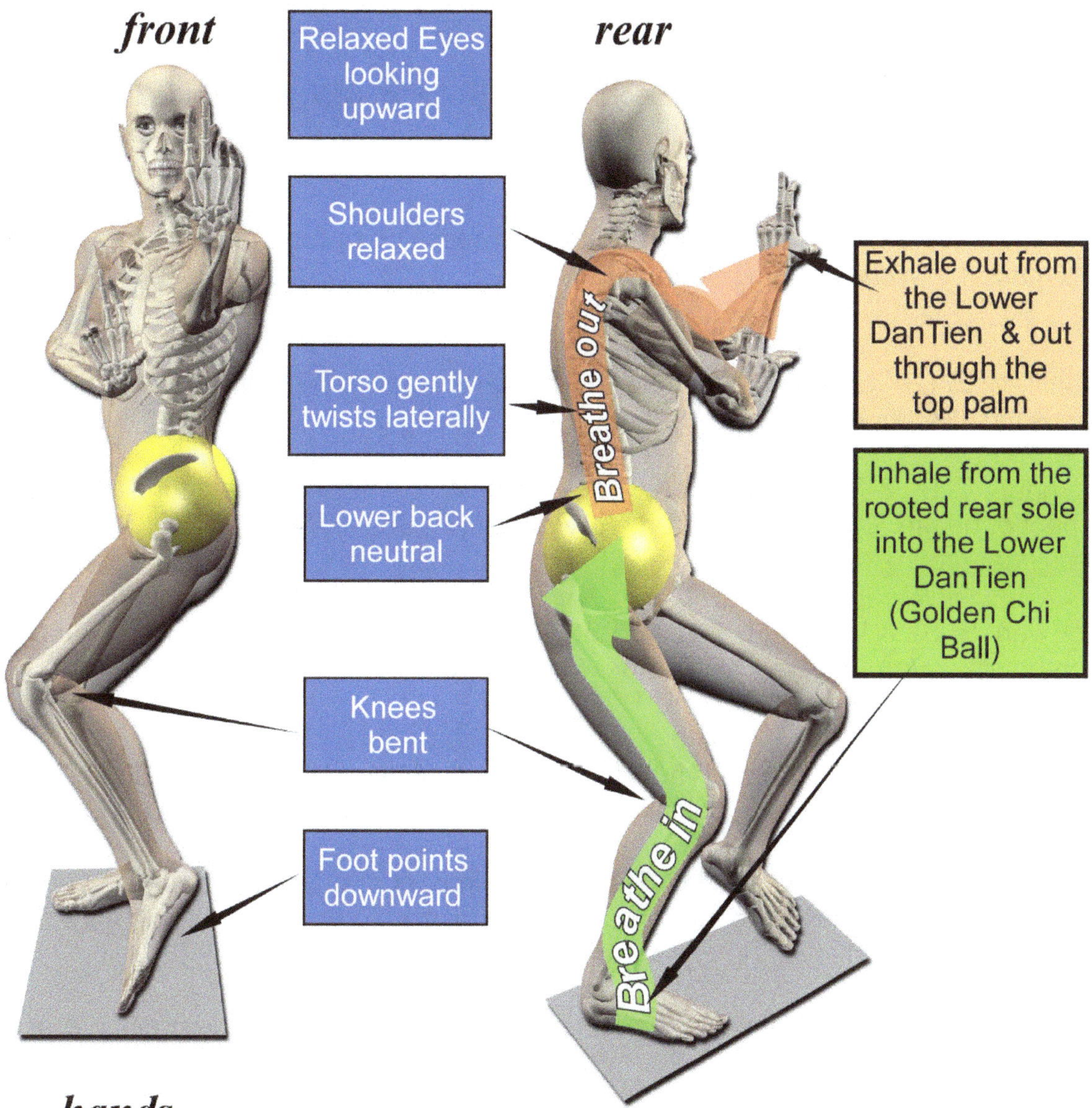

www.MindAndBodyExercises.com

front — Relaxed Eyes looking upward; Shoulders relaxed; Torso gently twists laterally; Lower back neutral; Knees bent; Foot points downward

rear — Exhale out from the Lower DanTien & out through the top palm; Inhale from the rooted rear sole into the Lower DanTien (Golden Chi Ball); Breathe Out; Breathe in

hands

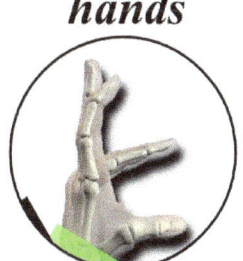

Set 8 stimulates the thrusting vessel while putting extra resistance on the wrists, thighs and ankles. Start with the feet, working your way up the body as applying the proper positions and posture. Inhale from upward palm down into the Lower DanTien. Exhale from this point and out through the sole of the rooted rear foot. Inhale from the sole into the DanTien. Exhale out from the DanTien and through the palm to complete 1 full repetition. Execute on both sides for 1 set.

REFERENCES — CHAPTER 7

Dienstbier, R. A. (1989). Arousal and physiological toughness: Implications for mental and physical health. *Psychological Review, 96*(1), 84–100. https://doi.org/10.1037/0033-295X.96.1.84

Dishman, R. K., Berthoud, H. R., Booth, F. W., Cotman, C. W., Edgerton, V. R., Fleshner, M. R., … Zigmond, M. J. (2006). Neurobiology of exercise. *Obesity, 14*(3), 345–356. https://doi.org/10.1038/oby.2006.46

Foa, E. B., & Kozak, M. J. (1986). Emotional processing of fear: Exposure to corrective information. *Psychological Bulletin, 99*(1), 20–35. https://doi.org/10.1037/0033-2909.99.1.20

Frankl, V. E. (2006). *Man's search for meaning* (Rev. ed.). Beacon Press. (Original work published 1946)

Kashdan, T. B., & Rottenberg, J. (2010). Psychological flexibility as a fundamental aspect of health. *Clinical Psychology Review, 30*(7), 865–878. https://doi.org/10.1016/j.cpr.2010.03.001

McEwen, B. S., & Wingfield, J. C. (2003). The concept of allostasis in biology and biomedicine. *Hormones and Behavior, 43*(1), 2–15. https://doi.org/10.1016/S0018-506X(02)00024-7

Porges, S. W. (2011). The polyvagal theory: Neurophysiological foundations of emotions, attachment, communication, and self-regulation. W. W. Norton & Company.

Ratey, J. J., & Loehr, J. E. (2011). The positive impact of physical activity on cognition during adulthood: A review of underlying mechanisms. *Exercise and Sport Sciences Reviews, 39*(4), 171–179. https://doi.org/10.1097/JES.0b013e31822d0a6c

Siegel, D. J. (2012). The developing mind: How relationships and the brain interact to shape who we are (2nd ed.). Guilford Press.

Southwick, S. M., Bonanno, G. A., Masten, A. S., Panter-Brick, C., & Yehuda, R. (2014). Resilience definitions, theory, and challenges. *European Journal of Psychotraumatology, 5*, 25338. https://doi.org/10.3402/ejpt.v5.25338

Tedeschi, R. G., & Calhoun, L. G. (2018). Posttraumatic growth: Theory, research, and applications. Routledge.

van der Kolk, B. A. (2014). The body keeps the score: Brain, mind, and body in the healing of trauma. Viking.

Part III — Identity, Meaning, and Psychological Integration

Chapter 8 - Boundaries, Discernment, and Psychological Autonomy

Trauma does not only injure the nervous system and emotional life. It often damages a person's **capacity for boundaries, self-trust, and autonomous decision-making**. Survivors may struggle to say no, tolerate mistreatment, over-accommodate others, submit to authority without discernment, or silence their own needs out of fear of conflict or abandonment. These are not personality flaws. They are adaptive survival strategies learned in unsafe environments (Herman, 1992; van der Kolk, 2014).

Post-traumatic growth requires more than emotional regulation and resilience. It requires the **reconstruction of psychological autonomy**, the ability to define one's inner and outer limits, evaluate influence accurately, and act from self-directed values rather than fear or conditioning.

Trauma and the Erosion of Boundaries

Boundaries are the invisible lines that define where one person ends and another begins physically, emotionally, cognitively, and morally. Healthy boundaries allow for connection without self-betrayal. Trauma disrupts this capacity through:

- Chronic violation
- Emotional neglect
- Enmeshment
- Coercion
- Betrayal
- Punishment for self-expression

(Herman, 1992).

When boundaries are repeatedly violated, individuals often adapt by becoming:

- Hyper-compliant
- Conflict-avoidant
- Emotionally self-sacrificing
- Over-responsible for others
- Unable to recognize personal limits

These adaptations reduce immediate danger but produce long-term psychological vulnerability.

Psychological Autonomy and Self-Authorship

Psychological autonomy refers to the ability to:

- Think independently
- Feel without suppression
- Evaluate reality accurately
- Make self-directed choices
- Hold personal values
- Tolerate disagreement
- Maintain internal authority

(Self-determination theory; Deci & Ryan, 2000).

Trauma undermines autonomy by teaching the nervous system that self-assertion leads to danger. As a result, survivors may unconsciously hand authority over to partners, leaders, institutions, ideologies, or social approval. Recovery restores the internal locus of control.

Post-traumatic growth requires not only healing from harm, but reclaiming ownership of the self.

Discernment Versus Compliance

Discernment is the capacity to accurately evaluate:

- Intent
- Power dynamics
- Psychological manipulation
- Emotional coercion
- Gaslighting
- Exploitation
- Narrative control

Trauma weakens discernment by activating fear-based thinking. When fear dominates, individuals may comply simply to remain safe, regardless of reality (Lifton, 1989; Herman, 1992).

Compliance without discernment is not moral virtue. It is a trauma response. Growth requires the capacity to ask:

- "Is this true?"
- "Is this ethical?"
- "Is this aligned with my values?"

- "Do I consent to this?"

Without discernment, autonomy cannot stabilize.

High-Control Environments and Boundary Collapse

Research on coercive systems, abusive relationships, and cultic groups shows that **boundary erosion is a central mechanism of psychological control** (Lifton, 1989; Singer, 2003). These systems often:

- Undermine critical thinking
- Redefine personal identity
- Restrict independent relationships
- Exploit guilt and fear
- Demand loyalty at the expense of self
- Punish dissent

Survivors exiting such systems often experience:

- Confusion
- Moral disorientation
- Guilt without clear cause
- Fear of independent thought
- Identity diffusion

Psychological autonomy must be rebuilt deliberately in these cases.

Boundaries as a Neurobiological Capacity

Boundaries are not merely cognitive concepts. They reflect **nervous system regulation**. A dysregulated nervous system struggles to detect threat accurately and oscillates between submission and defense. As regulation improves, individuals regain:

- Threat discrimination
- Tolerance of tension
- Assertive capacity
- Emotional containment
- Decision confidence

(Porges, 2011; Siegel, 2012).

Thus, boundary restoration depends directly on the somatic and emotional regulation capacities developed in earlier chapters.

The Emotional Cost of Boundary Violations

Repeated boundary violations produce:

- Chronic shame
- Learned helplessness
- Moral injury
- Self-abandonment
- Identity fragmentation

(Mollica, 2006; Herman, 1992).

Survivors may internalize the belief that their needs are dangerous, selfish, or invalid. This belief is one of the most deeply damaging legacies of trauma. Growth requires the reversal of this conditioning.

Relearning the Language of "No"

For many trauma survivors, learning to say **no** is one of the most difficult and transformative recovery tasks. Saying no activates:

- Fear of abandonment
- Fear of retaliation
- Fear of guilt
- Fear of being seen as "bad"

Yet no is not cruelty. It is **self-definition**. It is how individuals mark the borders of their identity.

Each time a survivor sets a boundary and remains safe afterward, the nervous system updates its threat model. Over time, self-assertion becomes tolerable, then natural.

Boundaries and Ethical Development

Psychological autonomy is inseparable from ethical maturity. When individuals cannot choose freely, morality collapses into obedience. When individuals regain autonomy, ethics become consciously chosen commitments rather than imposed rules.

Autonomy allows individuals to act from:

- Personal values
- Informed consent
- Moral discernment
- Responsibility rather than fear

This shift is a central marker for post-traumatic growth.

Relational Boundaries and Attachment Repair

Trauma disrupts attachment by teaching either:

- "Others are dangerous."
- "I must abandon myself to stay connected."

Healthy boundaries correct both distortions. They allow connection without submission and independence without isolation. Secure attachment emerges when individuals can maintain selfhood within relationship (Siegel, 2012).

From Boundarylessness to Self-Defined Identity

As survivors rebuild boundaries, they often experience a profound identity shift:

- From object → subject
- From role → self
- From obedience → authorship
- From fear → clarity

This shift is not selfish. It is the restoration of psychological adulthood.

Boundaries as the Architecture of Freedom

Without boundaries, freedom collapses into chaos or exploitation. With boundaries, freedom becomes structured, sustainable, and ethical. Boundaries protect:

- Energy

- Time
- Values
- Emotional health
- Physical safety
- Moral integrity

They allow growth without self-destruction.

Psychological Autonomy as a Pillar of Post-Traumatic Growth

Post-traumatic growth does not simply mean feeling better. It means becoming **self-directed, ethically grounded, and psychologically sovereign**. Survivors begin to experience:

- Confidence in perception
- Trust in decision-making
- Clear relational limits
- Reduced susceptibility to manipulation
- Stable identity across contexts

These changes reflect not symptom reduction, but structural psychological transformation.

From Survival Submission to Conscious Self-Direction

Trauma teaches submission for survival. Growth teaches self-direction for life. The same nervous system that once learned to comply now learns to choose. The same mind that once feared judgment now discerns truth. The same self that once dissolved now stands defined.

This is not rebellion. It is recovery.

REFERENCES — CHAPTER 8

Deci, E. L., & Ryan, R. M. (2000). The "what" and "why" of goal pursuits: Human needs and the self-determination of behavior. *Psychological Inquiry, 11*(4), 227–268. https://doi.org/10.1207/S15327965PLI1104_01

Herman, J. L. (1992). Trauma and recovery: The aftermath of violence—from domestic abuse to political terror. Basic Books.

Lifton, R. J. (1989). Thought reform and the psychology of totalism: A study of brainwashing in China. University of North Carolina Press.

Mollica, R. F. (2006). Healing invisible wounds: Paths to hope and recovery in a violent world. Harcourt.

Porges, S. W. (2011). The polyvagal theory: Neurophysiological foundations of emotions, attachment, communication, and self-regulation. W. W. Norton & Company.

Siegel, D. J. (2012). The developing mind: How relationships and the brain interact to shape who we are (2nd ed.). Guilford Press.

Singer, M. T. (2003). Cults in our midst: The continuing fight against their hidden menace (Revised ed.). Jossey-Bass.

van der Kolk, B. A. (2014). The body keeps the score: Brain, mind, and body in the healing of trauma. Viking.

Chapter 9 - Meaning-Making, Purpose, and Identity Reconstruction After Trauma

Trauma shatters assumptions. It fractures the framework through which people understand themselves, others, and the world. Beliefs once taken for granted, about safety, fairness, identity, morality, control, and meaning are suddenly disrupted or destroyed. This "shattering" is a hallmark of traumatic experience (Janoff-Bulman, 1992). When the world no longer makes sense, the mind is compelled to rebuild a new map of reality.

Post-traumatic growth occurs not *despite* this disruption, but *through it*. **Meaning-making** is the process by which survivors reconstruct their worldview, their purpose, and ultimately their own identity. This reconstruction is not a return to who they were before trauma, but the formation of a new, more coherent, more resilient self (Tedeschi & Calhoun, 2018).

The Collapse of Core Assumptions

Trauma destabilizes foundational beliefs:

- "The world is predictable."
- "I am safe."
- "People can be trusted."
- "I am in control of my life."
- "Bad things won't happen to me."

Such disruptions generate existential shock, leaving survivors to navigate confusion, grief, fear, and disorientation. This collapse is not a failure of character, but rather it is a normal cognitive response to abnormal circumstances (Janoff-Bulman, 1992; Park, 2010).

Yet this destabilization also creates a rare psychological opening: the potential to rebuild one's worldview on more grounded, realistic, and meaningful foundations.

Meaning-Making as a Healing Mechanism

Meaning-making refers to the process of interpreting trauma in ways that restore coherence and direction. It includes:

- Understanding the impact of the trauma
- Identifying what was violated or lost

- Integrating emotional experiences
- Creating a narrative that honors truth without collapse
- Discovering new values, strengths, or priorities

(Park, 2010; Tedeschi & Calhoun, 2004).

Meaning-making is not the search for a silver lining. It is the search for orientation, the rebuilding of a coherent inner world.

Why Meaning-Making Is Essential for PTG

Without meaning, trauma is experienced as random suffering. With meaning, suffering becomes transformed and not justified, but integrated.

Research shows that meaning-making:

- Reduces PTSD symptoms
- Strengthens emotional regulation
- Improves resilience
- Enhances psychological well-being
- Predicts long-term post-traumatic growth

(Park, 2010; Triplett et al., 2012).

Meaning is not given. It is constructed through reflection, engagement, and emotional processing.

Identity Disruption and Identity Development

Trauma destabilizes identity by introducing:

- Self-doubt
- Shame
- Disorientation
- Disconnection from values
- Fragmented self-narrative

(Neimeyer, 2019).

Identity reconstruction requires survivors to integrate the trauma into their life story in a way that does not define them but informs them. PTG does not frame trauma as destiny, but as a chapter that reshapes the trajectory of personal development.

Narrative Reconstruction: Rewriting the Self-Story

Narrative psychology shows that humans make sense of life through story. Trauma interrupts this story; meaning-making restores it. Narrative reconstruction involves:

- Placing the trauma in context
- Identifying its emotional and relational consequences
- Recognizing survival and resilience
- Making sense of the lessons or values that emerged
- Reframing identity in light of the new understanding

(Pennebaker & Smyth, 2016; Neimeyer, 2019).

The goal is not to glorify suffering but to create a coherent narrative that reflects truth, agency, and possibility.

The Role of Values in Purpose Reconstruction

Values act as internal guideposts. Trauma often causes people to lose sight of these guideposts or abandon them entirely in the wake of helplessness. Purpose reconstruction requires survivors to:

- Identify what matters most
- Distinguish inherited values from chosen ones
- Re-establish priorities
- Align action with meaning

Deci and Ryan's Self-Determination Theory emphasizes that autonomy, competence, and relatedness are crucial to intrinsic motivation and purpose (Deci & Ryan, 2000). Trauma disrupts these needs; PTG re-establishes them.

Discovering New Purpose Through Trauma

Many survivors report profound shifts in purpose as a result of trauma, including:

- Increased desire to help others
- Greater emphasis on relationships
- Renewed appreciation of life
- Heightened sense of spiritual or existential meaning
- Stronger personal mission or service orientation

(Tedeschi & Calhoun, 2018).

This is not universal nor is it required, but when it occurs, purpose becomes a stabilizing force in identity reconstruction.

Meaning-Making and Moral Injury

In cases where trauma involves betrayal, injustice, coercion, or violations of personal ethics, survivors may develop **moral injury,** a deep sense of guilt, shame, or disillusionment (Litz et al., 2009). Meaning-making in these cases focuses on:

- Understanding systemic or situational influences
- Separating responsibility from self-condemnation
- Reconstructing a moral identity
- Restoring integrity

This process is essential for those who have experienced complex trauma, institutional betrayal, or high-control environments.

The Emergence of the "New Self"

Identity reconstruction after trauma involves five key developments:

1. **Recognition** – acknowledging the ways trauma changed one's worldview
2. **Integration** – linking trauma into the life narrative without fragmentation
3. **Reorientation** – shifting values, priorities, and commitments
4. **Expansion** – developing new capabilities and perspectives
5. **Self-authorship** – choosing one's identity consciously rather than reactively

This process transforms survivors from passive recipients of life events into active authors of their future.

Meaning as a Core Feature of Post-Traumatic Growth

Meaning-making and purpose reconstruction represent two of the five major domains of PTG identified in the research:

- Appreciation of life
- Enhanced relationships
- Personal strength

- New possibilities
- Spiritual or existential growth

(Tedeschi & Calhoun, 2018).

Meaning acts as the integrating force across all these domains.

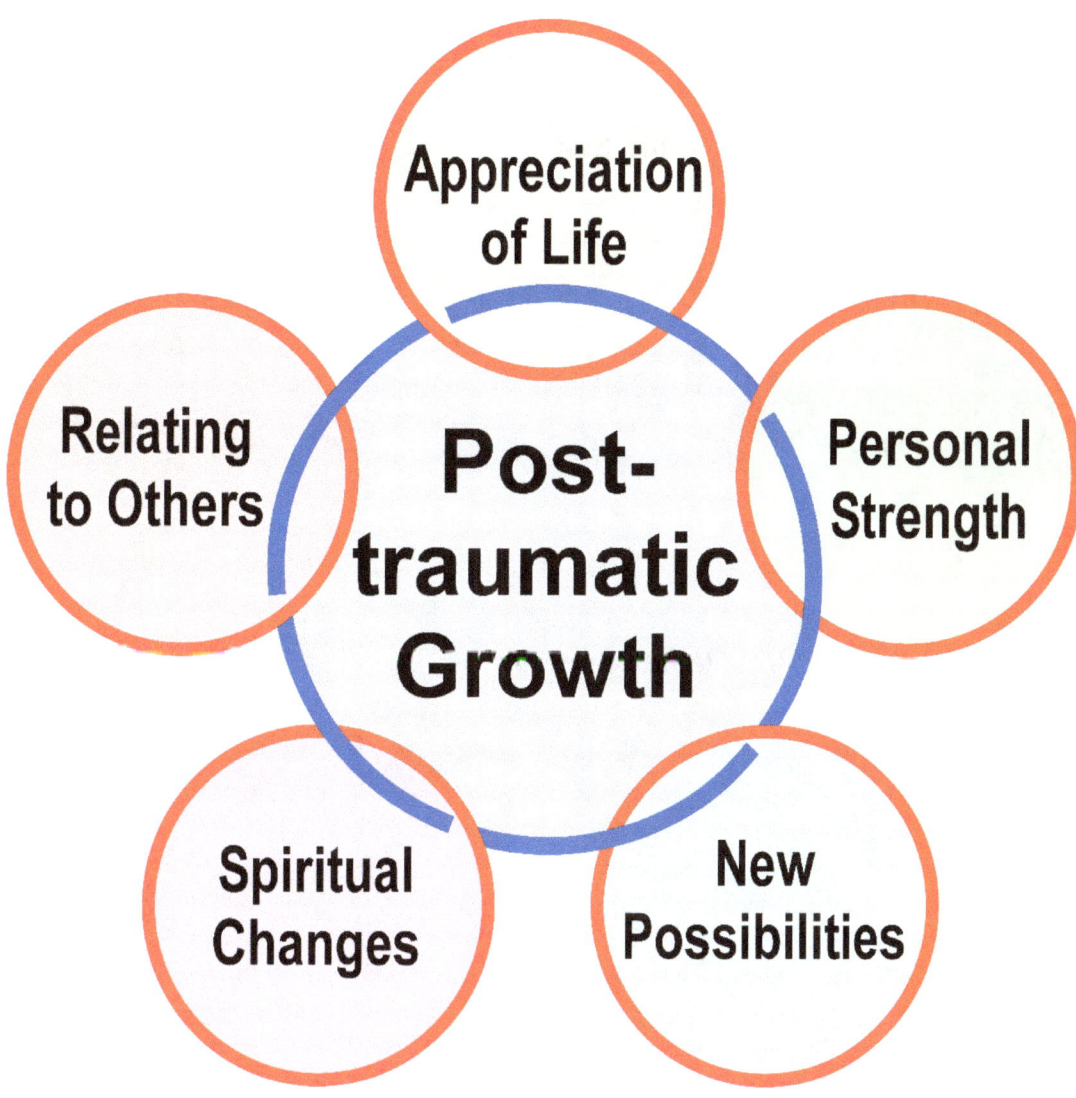

From Shattered Assumptions to Chosen Foundations

Trauma breaks the old foundations. Growth builds new ones. Meaning-making does not erase pain or minimize injustice. Instead, it transforms confusion into clarity, fragmentation into coherence, and despair into direction.

Survivors begin to say:

- "This experience changed me."
- "But I choose what that change means."
- "And I choose who I become because of it."

This is the essence of identity reconstruction.

Purpose as the Engine of the Future Self

When purpose emerges, survivors gain:

- Direction
- Motivation
- Stability
- Psychological resilience
- A reason to move forward

Purpose becomes the engine that drives the reconstructed identity into the future.

The trauma is no longer the center of the story. The person is.

REFERENCES — CHAPTER 9

Deci, E. L., & Ryan, R. M. (2000). The "what" and "why" of goal pursuits: Human needs and the self-determination of behavior. *Psychological Inquiry, 11*(4), 227–268. https://doi.org/10.1207/S15327965PLI1104_01

Janoff-Bulman, R. (1992). Shattered assumptions: Toward a new psychology of trauma. Free Press.

Litz, B. T., Stein, N., Delaney, E., Lebowitz, L., Nash, W., Silva, C., & Maguen, S. (2009). Moral injury and moral repair in war veterans. *Clinical Psychology Review, 29*(8), 695–706. https://doi.org/10.1016/j.cpr.2009.07.003

Neimeyer, R. A. (2019). Meaning reconstruction in grief and trauma: Foundations and applications. American Psychological Association.

Park, C. L. (2010). Making sense of the meaning literature: An integrative review of meaning making and its effects on adjustment to stressful life events. *Psychological Bulletin, 136*(2), 257–301. https://doi.org/10.1037/a0018301

Pennebaker, J. W., & Smyth, J. M. (2016). Opening up by writing it down: How expressive writing improves health and eases emotional pain (3rd ed.). Guilford Press.

Tedeschi, R. G., & Calhoun, L. G. (2004). Posttraumatic growth: Conceptual foundations and empirical evidence. *Psychological Inquiry, 15*(1), 1–18. https://doi.org/10.1207/s15327965pli1501_01

Tedeschi, R. G., & Calhoun, L. G. (2018). Posttraumatic growth: Theory, research, and applications. Routledge.

Triplett, K. N., Tedeschi, R. G., Cann, A., Calhoun, L. G., & Reeve, C. L. (2012). Posttraumatic growth, meaning in life, and life satisfaction in response to trauma. *Psychological Trauma: Theory, Research, Practice, and Policy, 4*(4), 400–410. https://doi.org/10.1037/a0024204

van der Kolk, B. A. (2014). The body keeps the score: Brain, mind, and body in the healing of trauma. Viking.

Chapter 10 - Shadow Work, Emotional Maturity, and Post-Traumatic Growth

Trauma leaves behind more than memories and nervous system imprints. It shapes internal patterns of perception, emotion, and behavior that often operate outside conscious awareness. These hidden patterns, sometimes called the "shadow," consist of the parts of ourselves we learned to suppress, deny, or exile in order to survive. In psychological terms, the shadow includes shame, fear, anger, mistrust, unresolved grief, defensive reactions, distorted beliefs, and internalized messages from abusive or invalidating environments (Herman, 1992; van der Kolk, 2014).

Shadow work is the process of bringing these unconscious patterns into awareness with compassion and curiosity. It is not a mystical exploration of darkness. It is the **integration of disowned emotional material** and the development of emotional maturity through honesty, reflection, and relational repair.

Post-traumatic growth requires this level of inner work. Without integrating shadow material, survivors may regulate their bodies and develop cognitive clarity—but still find themselves repeating patterns of sabotage, avoidance, defensiveness, or self-doubt.

Shadow work is the bridge between surviving trauma and transforming because of it.

The Shadow as a Survival Adaptation

The shadow forms as a protective mechanism. When emotions, reactions, or needs were unsafe in childhood or during traumatic periods, survivors learned to suppress them. Patterns often include:

- Anger turned inward because expression led to punishment
- Fear masked by rigidity or control
- Sadness buried beneath numbness
- Shame hidden behind perfectionism or compliance
- Needs suppressed to prevent abandonment

These suppressed parts do not disappear; they remain active in the nervous system and emotional memory networks (LeDoux, 2012). They resurface through:

- Overreactions
- Withdrawal
- Relationship conflict
- Self-criticism
- Projection onto others

- Shame spirals

Shadow work reveals these patterns not as moral failings, but as adaptive responses that once kept the survivor safe.

Emotional Maturity: Moving Beyond Defensive Patterns

Trauma often locks individuals into emotional survival strategies developed at earlier stages of life. Emotional maturity involves outgrowing these patterns and replacing them with more flexible, regulated responses (Siegel, 2012). Core markers of emotional immaturity rooted in trauma can include:

- Black-and-white thinking
- Difficulty tolerating discomfort
- Shame-based self-evaluation
- Externalizing blame
- Avoidance of conflict
- Suppression of anger or grief
- Hyper-reactivity to perceived criticism
- Dependency on external validation

Emotional maturity develops when survivors build the capacity to:

- Feel emotions without collapse
- Reflect before reacting
- Tolerate disagreement and complexity
- Hold oneself accountable without self-shaming
- Navigate conflict ethically
- Express needs without fear
- Repair relational ruptures

This maturation is a developmental process, not a personality change.

The Role of Emotional Honesty in Growth

Emotional honesty means acknowledging internal experiences without minimizing, denying, or rationalizing them. Survivors of trauma often learned to hide their internal world to avoid punishment or to maintain attachment relationships (Herman, 1992). As adults, this may manifest as:

- Pretending to be "fine" when overwhelmed
- Smiling through distress
- Hiding anger or hurt to avoid conflict
- Not expressing needs or preferences
- Agreeing externally while disagreeing internally

Emotional honesty reopens the possibility for self-connection and relational trust. Through honest recognition such as thinking "I am scared," "I am angry," "I feel unworthy," survivors reclaim parts of the self that were exiled.

Shame as the Core of the Shadow

Shame is one of the deepest emotional scars of trauma. Unlike guilt (a response to behavior), shame targets the self: "I am defective." Shame often fuels:

- Perfectionism
- Avoidance
- Rage
- Emotional withdrawal
- Relationship sabotage
- Imposter syndrome
- Deep self-criticism

(Tangney & Dearing, 2002; Neff, 2011).

Shadow work involves confronting shame not with judgment but with self-compassion. Research consistently shows that self-compassion reduces shame, increases emotional resilience, and supports adaptive emotional regulation (Neff, 2011).

Projection: Seeing the Shadow in Others

Projection is a psychological process in which individuals attribute disowned parts of themselves onto others. For trauma survivors, projection often arises when:

- Boundaries feel threatening
- Intimacy feels unsafe
- Authority triggers past dynamics
- Shame is activated
- Emotional needs conflict with conditioned self-erasure

Example:
A survivor may accuse a partner of anger or judgment when, in reality, the survivor fears their own anger or self-criticism.

Recognizing projection is an advanced form of emotional maturity. It enables individuals to distinguish:

- Past from present
- Internal from external
- Perception from reality

This clarity reduces relational conflict and restores agency.

Shadow Work and Moral Development

Trauma often leads to moral injury as deep wounds to one's sense of right, wrong, and self-worth when people are harmed, betrayed, coerced, or forced to violate their values (Litz et al., 2009). Shadow work includes:

- Acknowledging harm done to oneself
- Acknowledging harm done to others
- Processing guilt without collapsing into shame
- Restoring integrity
- Rebuilding an ethical self-identity

This is not confession; it is integration. Survivors reclaim themselves not as victims or perpetrators, but as evolving humans capable of repair, accountability, and growth.

Trauma, Reactivity, and the Shadow of Unmet Needs

Behind many trauma-driven behaviors lie unmet needs such as:

- Safety
- Security
- Belonging
- Recognition
- Autonomy
- Respect
- Boundaries
- Emotional validation

Unintegrated needs manifest through:

- Controlling behavior
- Avoidance of intimacy
- Rage
- Clinging
- Emotional withdrawal
- People-pleasing
- Overfunctioning or underfunctioning
- Perfectionism

Shadow work reveals these behaviors as messages, not malfunctions. When survivors meet these needs consciously, destructive patterns lose their power.

Integration: Turning Shadows into Strengths

Integration is the final step of shadow work. It involves bringing rejected emotions and patterns into conscious awareness and transforming them into mature psychological strengths.

Examples of integration:

- Suppressed anger → assertiveness and boundary protection
- Dissociation → present-moment awareness
- Shame → humility and compassion
- Hypervigilance → discernment
- Emotional sensitivity → empathy and relational attunement
- Rigidity → ethical clarity and consistency

Integrated shadow material becomes part of a stable, mature identity rather than an intrusive force.

Shadow Work and Post-Traumatic Growth

Post-traumatic growth researchers identify emotional maturity, personal strength, deeper relationships, and enhanced appreciation of life as core domains of long-term transformation (Tedeschi & Calhoun, 2018). Shadow work supports these domains by enabling survivors to:

- Take responsibility without self-condemnation

- Build emotional range
- Deepen relational capacity
- Develop ethical consistency
- Honor the truth of their experience
- Align behavior with values
- Live with authenticity rather than performance

Healing becomes not a return to who they were, but an emergence of who they have the capacity to become.

Shadow Work as a Lifelong Process

Integration is not a one-time event. It is a lifelong practice of:

- Self-reflection
- Emotional regulation
- Compassionate honesty
- Boundary maintenance
- Courageous dialogue
- Accountability
- Curiosity about one's own reactions

As survivors continue to engage with their shadow, they expand emotional maturity and deepen their sense of wholeness. Growth becomes continuous.

From Fragmentation to Wholeness

Trauma fragments the self. Shadow work reunites it. By bringing hidden material into conscious awareness with gentleness rather than judgment, survivors reclaim their full emotional, moral, and relational capacity. This integrated self is capable of:

- More stable relationships
- Clearer purpose
- Stronger boundaries
- Emotional resilience
- Ethical living
- Compassion for self and others

Shadow work transforms the survivor from someone shaped by trauma to someone shaped by integration, maturity, and freedom.

REFERENCES — CHAPTER 10

Herman, J. L. (1992). Trauma and recovery: The aftermath of violence—from domestic abuse to political terror. Basic Books.

LeDoux, J. E. (2012). *Rethinking the emotional brain. Neuron, 73*(4), 653–676. https://doi.org/10.1016/j.neuron.2012.02.004

Litz, B. T., Stein, N., Delaney, E., Lebowitz, L., Nash, W., Silva, C., & Maguen, S. (2009). Moral injury and moral repair in war veterans. *Clinical Psychology Review, 29*(8), 695–706. https://doi.org/10.1016/j.cpr.2009.07.003

Neff, K. D. (2011). Self-compassion: The proven power of being kind to yourself. William Morrow.

Siegel, D. J. (2012). The developing mind: How relationships and the brain interact to shape who we are (2nd ed.). Guilford Press.

Tangney, J. P., & Dearing, R. L. (2002). *Shame and guilt*. Guilford Press.

Tedeschi, R. G., & Calhoun, L. G. (2018). Posttraumatic growth: Theory, research, and applications. Routledge.

van der Kolk, B. A. (2014). The body keeps the score: Brain, mind, and body in the healing of trauma. Viking.

Chapter 11 - Conflict, Attachment Triggers, and Relational Healing

Trauma is never purely intrapsychic. It unfolds within relationships and leaves its deepest imprints there. Survivors often report that the greatest challenges in recovery are not panic attacks, intrusive memories, or physiological symptoms alone—but conflict, emotional reactivity, fear of abandonment, mistrust, and relational instability. These struggles are not character defects. They are the legacy of attachment injuries and threat-conditioned nervous systems (Herman, 1992; van der Kolk, 2014).

Post-traumatic growth is not complete until it extends into the relational field.

Growth must become lived within connection, not merely practiced in isolation.

Attachment as the Nervous System's Relational Blueprint

Attachment theory demonstrates that early relational experiences shape:

- Emotional regulation
- Threat perception
- Trust formation
- Boundary development
- Conflict response
- Intimacy tolerance

(Bowlby, 1988; Mikulincer & Shaver, 2016).

Trauma disrupts these systems by teaching the nervous system that proximity equals danger, abandonment, domination, or unpredictability. As a result, survivors may develop insecure attachment patterns:

- **Anxious attachment** — fear of abandonment, hypervigilance to rejection
- **Avoidant attachment** — emotional distancing, fear of dependence
- **Disorganized attachment** — oscillation between closeness and fear

These patterns are neurobiological adaptations, not conscious strategies.

Relational Triggers and the Reenactment of Trauma

A relational trigger is any interaction that activates unresolved survival circuitry. Common triggers include:

- Tone of voice

- Facial expression
- Perceived rejection
- Power imbalance
- Criticism
- Emotional withdrawal
- Assertive boundaries

When triggered, the nervous system reacts as if the original trauma is happening again. Individuals may respond with:

- Defensiveness
- Withdrawal
- Attack
- Collapse
- Pleasing
- Emotional flooding

(van der Kolk, 2014; Siegel, 2012).

These reactions are not deliberate. They are procedural memory responses stored in the body, not the cortex.

Conflict as a Mirror of Unhealed Attachment Wounds

In healthy systems, conflict is a signal for negotiation, repair, and growth. In trauma-conditioned systems, conflict becomes a perceived threat to survival. Survivors may experience:

- Terror of confrontation
- Explosive rage
- Dissociation during arguments
- Automatic submission
- Emotional shutdown

(Herman, 1992).

Conflict reveals not only current disagreement, but the nervous system's historical memory of danger. This is why minor disagreements can provoke disproportionate emotional reactions.

Shame and Defensive Reactivity in Relationships

Shame often becomes the hidden driver of relational conflict. When shame is activated, individuals may:

- Attack to protect against humiliation
- Withdraw to avoid exposure
- Blame others to escape self-condemnation
- Collapse into self-hatred

(Tangney & Dearing, 2002; Neff, 2011).

Relational healing requires the ability to recognize shame activation and regulate it rather than discharging it through attack or avoidance.

Neurobiology of Relational Safety

Relational safety depends on the **ventral vagal system**, which supports:

- Emotional attunement
- Facial expressiveness
- Vocal tone regulation
- Trust formation
- Empathy
- Co-regulation

(Porges, 2011).

Trauma dampens ventral vagal function and amplifies survival pathways. As nervous system regulation improves through breath, posture, and self-regulation (Chapters 2–6), relational capacity stabilizes accordingly. Relational healing is therefore inseparable from physiological regulation.

Co-Regulation and the Repair of Attachment

Co-regulation refers to the nervous system's ability to stabilize through safe connection. It develops through:

- Attuned listening
- Emotional validation
- Predictable responsiveness
- Respect for boundaries
- Repair after rupture

(Siegel, 2012; Mikulincer & Shaver, 2016).

For trauma survivors, co-regulation must be **relearned**. Many learned early that regulation was a solitary task or that others were unsafe. Growth involves discovering that stability can exist within relationship without self-abandonment.

Boundaries as Relational Stabilizers

Relational healing requires clear boundaries. Without boundaries, attachment becomes enmeshment, submission, or avoidance. With boundaries, connection becomes safe, voluntary, and mutual.

Boundaries allow individuals to:

- Remain emotionally present without collapse
- Express needs without fear
- Tolerate disagreement without rupture
- Repair conflict without domination
- Maintain identity within intimacy

(Deci & Ryan, 2000; Siegel, 2012).

This is not rigidity; it is relational integrity.

Repair After Rupture: The Central Skill of Mature Relationship

All relationships experience rupture. What distinguishes secure relationships is not the absence of conflict, but the **capacity for repair**. Repair involves:

- Acknowledgment of harm
- Regulation before dialogue
- Mutual perspective-taking
- Accountability without humiliation
- Restoration of trust

(Herman, 1992; Siegel, 2012).

For trauma survivors, repair is often terrifying because past ruptures led to abandonment, punishment, or annihilation.

Learning that rupture can be repaired, rather than feared, is a cornerstone of relational post-traumatic growth.

From Trauma Bonding to Secure Connection

Trauma bonding occurs when fear, reward, and attachment become fused within unsafe relationships. Survivors may equate intensity with intimacy and chaos with connection (van der Kolk, 2014).

Relational healing breaks this association and replaces it with:

- Stability without boredom
- Safety without submission
- Intimacy without annihilation
- Loyalty without self-betrayal

This transition reflects the maturation of the attachment system.

Relational Healing and Identity Reconstruction

As relationships stabilize, identity reorganizes. Survivors begin to experience themselves as:

- Worthy of respect
- Capable of mutuality
- Able to tolerate closeness
- Able to tolerate separation
- Able to maintain selfhood within connection

This identity shift is one of the most profound expressions of post-traumatic growth.

The Ethics of Relational Power

Trauma often involves power misuse through use of coercion, domination, silencing, or exploitation. Relational healing includes the development of **ethical power use**, defined by:

- Mutual consent
- Transparent influence
- Shared responsibility
- Non-coercion
- Accountability

This ethical awareness prevents the repetition of trauma dynamics within new relationships.

From Relational Survival to Relational Growth

In early recovery, relationships are often navigated through survival strategies. In post-traumatic growth, relationships become arenas for:

- Mutual development
- Emotional expansion
- Shared meaning
- Repair-based trust
- Ethical intimacy

Conflict no longer means annihilation. **It becomes the medium through which maturity develops**.

Relational Healing as a Central Domain of Post-Traumatic Growth

PTG research identifies improved relationships as one of the five core domains of growth:

- Deeper emotional intimacy
- Greater compassion
- Increased appreciation of others
- Enhanced relational commitment
- Stronger capacity for love

(Tedeschi & Calhoun, 2018).

Relational healing transforms trauma's greatest wound of disconnection into one of its deepest gifts: **authentic connection grounded in safety and choice**.

From Triggered Reaction to Conscious Relationship

Trauma teaches reaction. Growth teaches response. As survivors integrate their triggers, regulate their nervous systems, clarify boundaries, and repair ruptures, they step into relationships not as frightened children or armored defenders, but as conscious relational participants. This is not the end of conflict. It is the end of unconscious suffering within conflict.

REFERENCES — CHAPTER 11

Bowlby, J. (1988). A secure base: Parent-child attachment and healthy human development. Basic Books.

Deci, E. L., & Ryan, R. M. (2000). The "what" and "why" of goal pursuits: Human needs and the self-determination of behavior. *Psychological Inquiry, 11*(4), 227–268. https://doi.org/10.1207/S15327965PLI1104_01

Herman, J. L. (1992). Trauma and recovery: The aftermath of violence—from domestic abuse to political terror. Basic Books.

Mikulincer, M., & Shaver, P. R. (2016). *Attachment in adulthood: Structure, dynamics, and change* (2nd ed.). Guilford Press.

Neff, K. D. (2011). Self-compassion: The proven power of being kind to yourself. William Morrow.

Porges, S. W. (2011). The polyvagal theory: Neurophysiological foundations of emotions, attachment, communication, and self-regulation. W. W. Norton & Company.

Siegel, D. J. (2012). The developing mind: How relationships and the brain interact to shape who we are (2nd ed.). Guilford Press.

Tangney, J. P., & Dearing, R. L. (2002). *Shame and guilt*. Guilford Press.

Tedeschi, R. G., & Calhoun, L. G. (2018). Posttraumatic growth: Theory, research, and applications. Routledge.

van der Kolk, B. A. (2014). The body keeps the score: Brain, mind, and body in the healing of trauma. Viking.

Part IV — Growth, Contribution, and Life Reintegration

Chapter 12 - Expanded Self-Awareness and Psychological Maturity

Post-traumatic growth is not defined solely by symptom reduction, emotional regulation, or resilience under stress. At its deepest level, growth expresses itself as expanded self-awareness and psychological maturity. This represents the transition from survival-driven functioning into self-reflective, ethically grounded, and developmentally integrated adulthood.

Survivors begin to understand not only *what they feel,* but *why they feel it, how it shapes their behavior,* and *how their internal world affects others* (Siegel, 2012; Tedeschi & Calhoun, 2018).

Psychological maturity is not perfection. It is the ability to observe oneself honestly, tolerate emotional complexity, take responsibility without collapse, and live with increasing coherence between values, behavior, and identity.

From Reactive Consciousness to Reflective Awareness

Trauma organizes consciousness around immediacy and threat. Attention becomes reactive rather than reflective. The nervous system prioritizes rapid defense over contemplation, and behavior is driven by conditioned responses rather than conscious choice (van der Kolk, 2014).

Expanded self-awareness marks the shift from:

- Automatic reaction → intentional response
- Emotional flooding → emotional observation
- External blame → internal reflection
- Impulsive defense → regulated discernment

This shift depends on the strengthening of **prefrontal cortical regulation**, which supports introspection, impulse control, perspective-taking, and moral reasoning (Siegel, 2012).

Self-Awareness as an Executive Function

Self-awareness is not merely insight. It is a neurocognitive capacity involving:

- Interoceptive awareness (body-based perception)
- Emotional labeling
- Metacognitive reflection

- Pattern recognition
- Behavioral monitoring
- Ethical self-evaluation

(Menon, 2011; LeDoux, 2012).

Trauma disrupts these functions by fragmenting attention and suppressing reflective awareness. As regulation stabilizes and identity consolidates, these functions reintegrate into a coherent observing self.

Psychological Maturity as a Developmental Achievement

Psychological maturity involves the capacity to:

- Hold conflicting emotions without splitting
- Accept responsibility without excessive shame
- Tolerate frustration without collapse or rage
- Maintain identity during disagreement
- Regulate impulses ethically
- Maintain long-term perspective
- Balance self-interest with relational responsibility

This form of maturity does not arise automatically with age. It arises through developmental integration, often catalyzed by trauma and supported by intentional recovery work (Erikson, 1968; Siegel, 2012).

Trauma and Arrested Development

Trauma often arrests emotional development at the age or stage at which overwhelming threat occurred. Survivors may carry:

- Childlike fear responses
- Adolescent defiance or shame
- Rigid moral binaries
- Dependency or hyper-independence
- Avoidance of responsibility
- Emotional numbing

These patterns do not reflect immaturity of character. They reflect interrupted developmental processes. Psychological maturity involves re-entering and completing these stages consciously.

Metacognition and the Observer Self

One of the most reliable indicators of psychological maturity is **metacognition**, or the capacity to observe one's own thoughts, emotions, and behavior without being consumed by them (Teasdale et al., 2003).

With expanded awareness, survivors begin to notice:

- "This thought is familiar."
- "This reaction belongs to a past context."
- "This feeling is intense, but temporary."
- "This impulse does not require action."

This observer stance transforms identity from being fused with emotional states to being the container of experience rather than its prisoner.

Emotion Differentiation and Maturity

Trauma compresses emotional experience into extremes: fear or numbness, rage or collapse. Psychological maturity expands **emotion differentiation**, the ability to distinguish subtle emotional states such as:

- Anger vs. boundary violation
- Fear vs. uncertainty
- Grief vs. regret
- Guilt vs. shame
- Sadness vs. despair

Higher emotion differentiation is associated with greater emotional regulation, better relationships, and improved mental health outcomes (Kashdan et al., 2015).

Psychological Maturity and Ethical Self-Regulation

As self-awareness expands, ethical self-regulation strengthens. Survivors begin to:

- Anticipate the impact of their behavior on others
- Hold themselves accountable without humiliation
- Regulate impulses based on values rather than fear
- Distinguish responsibility from self-blame
- Choose restraint without repression

This reflects the maturation of the **moral self**, not through obedience, but through internalized ethical discernment (Erikson, 1968; Siegel, 2012).

Tolerance for Ambiguity and Complexity

Trauma drives the nervous system toward rigid certainty: safe/dangerous, good/bad, loyal/traitor. Psychological maturity restores the capacity to tolerate:

- Uncertainty
- Mixed motivations
- Conflicting emotions
- Imperfect choices
- Partial truths
- Gradual change

Cognitive flexibility and tolerance of ambiguity are core markers of adult psychological integration and resilience (Kashdan & Rottenberg, 2010).

Self-Awareness and Relational Maturity

Expanded self-awareness directly reshapes relationships. Survivors begin to:

- Recognize their own projections
- Identify emotional triggers in real time
- Pause before reacting
- Distinguish past from present
- Take responsibility for relational rupture
- Engage in repair without domination or collapse

This level of awareness allows relationships to become sites of co-development rather than reenactment (Siegel, 2012; Mikulincer & Shaver, 2016).

Identity Coherence and the Mature Self

As awareness expands, identity becomes more coherent. Survivors experience:

- Reduced internal fragmentation
- Increased consistency across roles

- Greater alignment between values and behavior
- Less dependence on external validation
- Greater tolerance of difference without identity threat

This coherence represents a core dimension of post-traumatic growth.

From Conditioned Self to Conscious Self

Psychological maturity reflects the shift from:

- Conditioned behavior → chosen behavior
- External authority → internal discernment
- Shame-driven compliance → value-driven action
- Emotional fusion → reflective agency

Survivors no longer live primarily from what was done to them, but from who they are becoming.

Expanded Self-Awareness as a Structural Transformation

Expanded self-awareness is not merely insight. It is a **structural reorganization of consciousness**. Survivors move from:

- Fragmentation → integration
- Reactivity → response
- Projection → ownership
- Collapse → reflection
- Survival → deliberate living

This marks the passage from trauma-driven identity to psychologically mature authorship of the self.

Psychological Maturity as a Pillar of Post-Traumatic Growth

Post-traumatic growth research consistently identifies psychological maturity as a central long-term outcome:

- Increased personal strength
- Emotional depth
- Ethical clarity
- Improved relationships
- Greater life appreciation
- Expanded existential perspective

(Tedeschi & Calhoun, 2018).

This is not superficial positivity. It is earned development through integration.

From Awareness to Responsibility

With expanded awareness comes responsibility not as burden, but as ownership of one's inner and outer life. Survivors recognize:

- "I did not choose what happened."
- "But I am choosing who I become."

This is the heart of psychological maturity.

REFERENCES — CHAPTER 12

Erikson, E. H. (1968). *Identity: Youth and crisis*. W. W. Norton & Company.

Kashdan, T. B., & Rottenberg, J. (2010). Psychological flexibility as a fundamental aspect of health. *Clinical Psychology Review, 30*(7), 865–878. https://doi.org/10.1016/j.cpr.2010.03.001

Kashdan, T. B., Barrett, L. F., & McKnight, P. E. (2015). Unpacking emotion differentiation: Transforming unpleasant experience by perceiving distinctions in negativity. *Current Directions in Psychological Science, 24*(1), 10–16. https://doi.org/10.1177/0963721414550708

LeDoux, J. E. (2012). *Rethinking the emotional brain. Neuron, 73*(4), 653–676. https://doi.org/10.1016/j.neuron.2012.02.004

Menon V. (2011). Large-scale brain networks and psychopathology: a unifying triple network model. *Trends in cognitive sciences*, *15*(10), 483–506. https://doi.org/10.1016/j.tics.2011.08.003

Mikulincer, M., & Shaver, P. R. (2016). *Attachment in adulthood: Structure, dynamics, and change* (2nd ed.). Guilford Press.

Siegel, D. J. (2012). The developing mind: How relationships and the brain interact to shape who we are (2nd ed.). Guilford Press.

Teasdale, J. D., Segal, Z. V., & Williams, J. M. G. (2003). Mindfulness training and problem formulation. *Clinical Psychology: Science and Practice, 10*(2), 157–160. https://doi.org/10.1093/clipsy.bpg017

Tedeschi, R. G., & Calhoun, L. G. (2018). Posttraumatic growth: Theory, research, and applications. Routledge.

van der Kolk, B. A. (2014). The body keeps the score: Brain, mind, and body in the healing of trauma. Viking.

Chapter 13 - Reclaiming Agency, Choice, and Life Direction

Trauma fundamentally disrupts the experience of agency. In moments of overwhelming threat, choice collapses, autonomy disappears, and behavior becomes governed by survival reflexes rather than intentional action. Long after the danger has passed, many survivors continue to live as if they have no real power over their circumstances. They may feel stuck, reactive, resigned, or dependent on external authority. This loss of agency is not weakness. It is the **neuropsychological imprint of uncontrollable stress** (Herman, 1992; van der Kolk, 2014).

Post-traumatic growth requires the restoration of agency, the lived experience of being able to choose, initiate, influence, and direct one's own life. Without agency, meaning cannot be enacted, boundaries cannot be sustained, identity cannot stabilize, and psychological maturity cannot fully emerge.

The Neurobiology of Helplessness

Repeated exposure to uncontrollable stress produces **learned helplessness**, a state marked by reduced motivation, impaired problem-solving, and emotional withdrawal (Maier & Seligman, 1976). Neurobiologically, helplessness is associated with:

- Reduced prefrontal regulation
- Heightened amygdala reactivity
- Suppressed dopaminergic motivation
- Impaired goal-directed behavior

(Maier & Seligman, 2016).

Trauma repeatedly teaches the nervous system: "Nothing I do changes the outcome." Post-traumatic growth directly reverses this imprint through experiences of effective action and recovery.

Agency as a Biological and Psychological Capacity

Agency is not merely a belief. It is a biological state supported by:

- Stable autonomic regulation
- Executive functioning
- Dopamine-based motivation
- Accurate threat discrimination
- Emotional self-regulation

(Porges, 2011; Schultz, 2016).

As the nervous system stabilizes and emotional maturity deepens (Chapters 10–12), the biological conditions for agency progressively return.

From Reaction to Response

Trauma conditions automatic reaction. Psychological maturity enables deliberate response. A reactive state is characterized by:

- Impulsivity
- Emotional flooding
- Avoidance
- Submission
- Defensiveness

A responsive state is characterized by:

- Pausing
- Evaluating
- Choosing
- Acting with intention
- Tolerating uncertainty

(Siegel, 2012).

Agency exists in the space between stimulus and response.

Self-Efficacy and the Restoration of Confidence

Self-efficacy refers to the belief that one can successfully influence outcomes through effort (Bandura, 1997). Trauma erodes this belief by pairing effort with failure, punishment, or humiliation.

Post-traumatic growth restores self-efficacy through:

- Gradual mastery experiences
- Boundary assertion with safe outcomes
- Regulation during emotional stress
- Follow-through on self-chosen commitments
- Successful navigation of challenge

Each completed act of agency strengthens confidence and rewires motivational circuitry.

Strategic Stress vs. Accidental Trauma: The Difference Between Chosen Challenge and Psychological Injury

Trauma, by definition, is uncontrollable, overwhelming, and disorganizing to the nervous system. It cannot be ethically prescribed or intentionally inflicted. However, growth-oriented disciplines across psychology, neuroscience, and rehabilitation consistently demonstrate that **voluntarily chosen, time-limited, and controlled stress** can strengthen agency rather than destroy it. For this reason, the more precise and ethically sound term is **strategic stress**.

Strategic stress refers to:

- Deliberate exposure to challenge
- Voluntary engagement with difficulty
- Stress experienced within a context of choice, meaning, and recovery

This distinction is critical. When challenge is chosen rather than imposed, it enhances **self-efficacy**, **internal locus of control**, and **adaptive learning**, the very mechanisms disrupted in traumatic helplessness (Bandura, 1997; Rotter, 1966; Maier & Seligman, 2016). Neurobiologically, controlled challenge engages dopamine-based learning systems that strengthen motivation, prediction, and behavioral flexibility (Schultz, 2016), while autonomic regulation supports physiological safety (Porges, 2011).

In contrast, **accidental trauma** strips the individual of agency, predictability, and control, core conditions for the development of learned helplessness (Maier & Seligman, 1976) and post-traumatic dysregulation (van der Kolk, 2014).

Within post-traumatic growth, strategic stress functions as **a recalibration of control after uncontrollable harm**. It is the process by which survivors gradually reclaim authorship over their nervous system, decisions, and identity, transforming helplessness into agency and suffering into strength (Tedeschi & Calhoun, 2018; Herman, 1992).

Disciplined practices of controlled stress training, such as the stance work introduced in Chapter 7, provide a direct neurological foundation for rebuilding agency, choice, and self-directed effort.

Choice as a Core Antidote to Trauma

Trauma is defined by the **loss of choice**. Recovery is defined by its return. Choice does not mean limitless control. It means:

- The capacity to consent
- The capacity to refuse
- The capacity to change direction
- The capacity to define priorities

Choice restores dignity and self-authorship.

Decision-Making After Trauma

Decision-making is commonly impaired after trauma due to:

- Fear of making mistakes
- Catastrophic thinking
- Dependence on authority
- Shame-based self-doubt
- Avoidance of responsibility

(van der Kolk, 2014; Herman, 1992).

Growth involves relearning how to decide, beginning with low-risk decisions and gradually expanding into larger life domains.

From External Control to Internal Locus of Control

Trauma often shifts locus of control outward. Survivors may feel that authority figures, institutions, or fate determine their lives. Post-traumatic growth re-establishes an **internal locus of control** (Rotter, 1966), which is associated with:

- Greater resilience
- Improved problem-solving
- Lower depression
- Higher life satisfaction

Agency does not eliminate uncertainty. It restores participation.

Agency and Identity Reconstruction

As agency returns, identity reorganizes. Survivors begin to experience themselves as:

- Actors rather than victims
- Contributors rather than burdens
- Decision-makers rather than dependents
- Adults rather than managed subjects

This identity transformation is a defining structural shift of post-traumatic growth.

Agency in the Face of Uncertainty

Agency does not require certainty. Trauma teaches that uncertainty equals danger. Growth teaches that uncertainty is an unavoidable condition of life. Agency allows individuals to act despite not knowing outcomes, grounded in values rather than fear.

Reclaiming Life Direction After Trauma

Trauma often ruptures life trajectory. Goals collapse. Motivation dissipates. The future becomes opaque. Reclaiming life direction involves:

- Establishing short-term goals
- Clarifying personal values
- Testing new possibilities
- Allowing identity to evolve
- Releasing pre-trauma expectations

Life direction after trauma is not a return to a previous path. It is the construction of a new trajectory informed by lived experience.

Agency and Responsibility

With agency comes responsibility not as burden, but as ownership. Survivors begin to recognize:

- "I did not choose what happened."
- "But I can choose what happens next."

This distinction protects against both self-blame and helplessness.

From Survival Obedience to Self-Directed Living

Trauma conditions obedience to danger cues, power structures, and fear-based authority. Post-traumatic growth restores self-directed living, guided by:

- Personal values
- Discernment
- Boundary clarity
- Emotional regulation
- Meaning

The survivor no longer lives primarily in reaction to the past, but in relationship to the future.

Agency as the Engine of Post-Traumatic Growth

Agency activates every other dimension of growth:

- Without agency, meaning remains abstract
- Without agency, resilience remains untested
- Without agency, boundaries collapse
- Without agency, relationships stagnate
- Without agency, identity fragments

With agency restored, growth becomes embodied and enacted.

From Helplessness to Participation

The deepest transformation of post-traumatic growth is the movement from:

- Helplessness → Participation
- Passivity → Initiative
- Reaction → Intention
- Fear → Choice
- Survival → Self-directed life

This is the reclamation of the survivor as an active author of their existence.

REFERENCES — CHAPTER 13

Bandura, A. (1997). Self-efficacy: The exercise of control. W. H. Freeman.

Herman, J. L. (1992). Trauma and recovery: The aftermath of violence—from domestic abuse to political terror. Basic Books.

Maier, S. F., & Seligman, M. E. P. (1976). Learned helplessness: Theory and evidence. *Journal of Experimental Psychology: General, 105*(1), 3–46. https://doi.org/10.1037/0096-3445.105.1.3

Maier, S. F., & Seligman, M. E. P. (2016). Learned helplessness at fifty: Insights from neuroscience. *Psychological Review, 123*(4), 349–367. https://doi.org/10.1037/rev0000033

Porges, S. W. (2011). The polyvagal theory: Neurophysiological foundations of emotions, attachment, communication, and self-regulation. W. W. Norton & Company.

Rotter, J. B. (1966). Generalized expectancies for internal versus external control of reinforcement. *Psychological Monographs: General and Applied, 80*(1), 1–28. https://doi.org/10.1037/h0092976

Schultz, W. (2016). Dopamine reward prediction-error signalling: A two-component response. *Nature Reviews Neuroscience, 17*(3), 183–195. https://doi.org/10.1038/nrn.2015.26

Siegel, D. J. (2012). The developing mind: How relationships and the brain interact to shape who we are (2nd ed.). Guilford Press.

Tedeschi, R. G., & Calhoun, L. G. (2018). Posttraumatic growth: Theory, research, and applications. Routledge.

van der Kolk, B. A. (2014). The body keeps the score: Brain, mind, and body in the healing of trauma. Viking.

Chapter 14 - Service, Contribution, and the Mature Expression of Growth

One of the most consistent findings in post-traumatic growth research is that individuals who move through the deep work of recovery often feel called to serve, guide, or support others. This shift does not arise from obligation but from a transformed understanding of suffering, resilience, and shared humanity (Tedeschi & Calhoun, 2018). When a survivor reaches this phase, growth becomes relational, generative, and socially expressed.

Service is not self-sacrifice. It is the mature expression of a self that has integrated pain into wisdom, boundaries into discernment, and agency into meaningful action. Contribution becomes the outward manifestation of inner coherence.

The Evolution of Motivation: From Survival to Generativity

Trauma forces the psyche to focus on immediate survival. As healing progresses, motivation gradually expands:

- From avoiding harm → to seeking stability
- From stability → to self-understanding
- From self-understanding → to autonomy and agency
- From agency → to purpose, belonging, and contribution

This developmental sequence mirrors Erikson's later-stage concept of **generativity**, the desire to contribute to the welfare of others and the next generation (Erikson, 1968).

In this stage of growth, survivors often feel:

- A deepened sense of responsibility
- Compassion for others who suffer
- Motivation to prevent harm where possible
- Desire to use hard-earned strengths for collective benefit
- A recognition that meaning grows when shared

Service becomes the next natural step in the recovery process.

Wisdom as the Product of Integrated Experience

True service arises from wisdom, not from unresolved wounds or savior impulses. Wisdom represents an integration of:

- Emotional maturity
- Empathy
- Discernment
- Boundary clarity
- Life experience
- Reflective self-awareness

(Linley, 2003; Siegel, 2012).

Survivors who have completed the earlier stages of growth possess a unique form of relational wisdom: they understand suffering without judgment, endurance without idealization, and healing without illusion.

Altruism Born of Suffering

Research shows that trauma can increase **prosocial motivation**, especially when survivors make meaning from their experience (Staub & Vollhardt, 2008). This phenomenon, sometimes called *altruism born of suffering,* emerges when individuals convert personal adversity into empathic concern and constructive action.

Examples include:

- Supporting others with similar traumatic histories
- Mentoring or teaching
- Community engagement
- Advocacy work
- Creative and educational contributions
- Preventative or protective efforts

In this phase, the survivor's life story becomes a source of guidance rather than a source of shame.

Compassion as a Mature Capacity

Compassion evolves as emotional defenses soften and self-awareness expands. It reflects the ability to:

- Recognize suffering
- Emotionally resonate without being overwhelmed
- Act ethically and responsibly
- Maintain boundaries while remaining open
- Extend care without self-erasure

(Neff, 2011).

Compassion is not sentimental. It is a regulated, grounded expression of connection that emerges from emotional stability and psychological maturity.

The Role of Boundaries in Mature Service

Healthy contribution requires boundaries. Without them, service becomes:

- Self-sacrifice
- Compulsion
- Role fusion
- Rescue behavior
- Burnout
- Identity loss

Survivors who have strengthened their boundaries (Chapter 8) can give from a place of choice rather than compulsion. They offer support without absorbing another's distress, and they maintain inner balance while remaining relationally available.

Boundaries make service sustainable.

Agency and Contribution: The Ethical Dimension of Growth

As agency develops (Chapter 13), individuals gain not only freedom but **ethical responsibility**. Mature agency includes:

- Awareness of the impact of one's actions
- Commitment to honesty and integrity
- Respect for others' autonomy
- Willingness to repair harm
- Engagement in community or relational systems

This is not moral perfection but ethical participation, living in a way that contributes rather than harms.

Trauma-Informed Contribution

A trauma-informed approach to service acknowledges:

- The universality of vulnerability
- The diversity of trauma responses
- The necessity of consent and autonomy
- The importance of safety, predictability, and respect
- The limits of one individual's role in another's healing

Survivors who embrace trauma-informed contribution avoid reenacting harmful dynamics such as coercion, dependency, or saviorism. Instead, they cultivate reciprocity and empowerment.

Creativity as Contribution

Many survivors find their contribution emerging through creative expression, including:

- Writing
- Art
- Movement (yoga, Pilates, dance, etc.)
- Martial arts
- Teaching
- Public speaking
- Music
- Wellness coaching
- Spiritual or philosophical reflection

Creativity transforms internal experience into shared meaning. It integrates identity, purpose, and expression are all hallmarks of mature post-traumatic growth.

Leadership as a Mature Expression of Growth

Leadership does not necessarily involve formal authority. Trauma-informed leadership expresses itself through:

- Integrity
- Consistency
- Emotional regulation
- Listening

- Purpose-driven action
- Ethical clarity
- Empathy without enmeshment

Leadership in this sense is the ability to influence through presence, values, and example, not dominance or control.

The Survivor as Mentor, Guide, or Example

Many trauma survivors become powerful mentors because they offer:

- Lived experience rather than abstract theory
- Compassion informed by suffering
- Stability informed by discipline
- Hope informed by personal transformation
- Boundaries informed by learned wisdom

This form of relational guidance is deeply impactful because it is authentic, grounded, and earned.

Contribution as Identity Integration

Contribution strengthens identity by linking personal history with present purpose. Survivors often experience:

- Increased meaning
- Reduced shame
- A sense of coherence
- A place within community
- A story that contributes rather than isolates

Identity shifts from "What happened to me?" to "What I bring into the world."

Service Without Self-Effacement: The Balance of Mature Growth

Mature contribution is balanced. Survivors learn to:

- Give without depletion
- Help without overidentifying
- Support without rescuing
- Lead without controlling
- Care without absorbing

This balance reflects the deeper integration of Chapters 8–13: boundaries, emotional maturity, agency, and expanded self-awareness.

Contribution as the Extension of Healing

Service is not the end of the healing journey, nor is it a requirement. But when it emerges naturally, it becomes a profound expression of:

- Integration
- Maturity
- Connection
- Purpose
- Ethical participation in life

Post-traumatic growth becomes generative when healing is no longer only inward but extends outward.

> *In this phase, the survivor becomes a source of stability and meaning for themselves and for others.*

REFERENCES — CHAPTER 14

Erikson, E. H. (1968). *Identity: Youth and crisis*. W. W. Norton & Company.

Linley P. A. (2003). Positive adaptation to trauma: wisdom as both process and outcome. *Journal of traumatic stress*, *16*(6), 601–610. https://doi.org/10.1023/B:JOTS.0000004086.64509.09

Neff, K. D. (2011). Self-compassion: The proven power of being kind to yourself. William Morrow.

Siegel, D. J. (2012). The developing mind: How relationships and the brain interact to shape who we are (2nd ed.). Guilford Press.

Staub, E., & Vollhardt, J. R. (2008). Altruism born of suffering: The roots of caring and helping after victimization and other trauma. *American Journal of Orthopsychiatry, 78*(3), 267–280. https://doi.org/10.1037/a0014223

Tedeschi, R. G., & Calhoun, L. G. (2018). Posttraumatic growth: Theory, research, and applications. Routledge.

van der Kolk, B. A. (2014). The body keeps the score: Brain, mind, and body in the healing of trauma. Viking.

Chapter 15 - Integration, Wholeness, and the Ongoing Growth Process

Post-traumatic growth is not a destination. It is not a fixed state of enlightenment, permanent peace, or completed transformation. It is a continuing process of integration, in which the body, mind, identity, relationships, and values are repeatedly reorganized around increasing levels of coherence, agency, and meaning. Wholeness does not mean that pain disappears. It means that pain no longer dominates perception, identity, or action (Tedeschi & Calhoun, 2018; Siegel, 2012).

This final chapter brings together the full arc of recovery explored throughout the book: from trauma and nervous system disruption, through emotional regulation and resilience, into identity reconstruction, agency, service, and ultimately a mature, integrated life orientation.

What Integration Truly Means

Integration refers to the linking of once-fragmented experience into a coherent whole. Trauma fragments:

- Memory
- Identity
- Affect
- Perception
- Bodily awareness
- Moral understanding
- Relational trust

(van der Kolk, 2014; Ogden et al., 2006).

Integration restores these into a coordinated system in which individuals can:

- Remember without reliving
- Feel without being overwhelmed
- Reflect without collapsing into shame
- Engage relationships without reenactment
- Hold identity without fragmentation

Wholeness is not perfection. It is functional coherence across domains of life.

The Body as a Foundation of Wholeness

Trauma embeds itself in the body through altered autonomic regulation, muscular bracing, breath restriction, and disrupted interoception (van der Kolk, 2014). Integration requires continued attention to:

- Breath regulation
- Postural integrity
- Movement-based self-regulation
- Grounding practices
- Sensory awareness

These are not preparatory tools that can be abandoned once insight is gained. They remain core stabilizers of the integrated self across the lifespan.

Psychological Integration and the Unified Self

Psychological integration involves the unification of:

- Thought
- Emotion
- Behavior
- Identity
- Moral reasoning
- Interpersonal functioning

(Siegel, 2012).

As integration deepens, survivors experience:

- Increased internal consistency
- Reduced compartmentalization
- Fewer abrupt state shifts
- Greater emotional fluidity
- Stable self-reference under stress

This unified self is capable of complexity without fragmentation and responsibility without collapse.

Relational Integration: From Wounding to Connection

Relational wholeness does not mean the absence of conflict. It means the capacity to:

- Tolerate rupture
- Engage in repair
- Maintain selfhood within intimacy
- Respect others' autonomy
- Hold boundaries without withdrawal or aggression

(Mikulincer & Shaver, 2016; Siegel, 2012).

Integrated relationships become sites of mutual development rather than reenactment of trauma dynamics. They engage as differentiated, responsible participants.

Survivors no longer seek salvation through others or isolate themselves in fear.

Moral Integration and Ethical Coherence

Trauma often fractures moral identity through betrayal, coercion, and injustice. Integration restores moral coherence by allowing survivors to:

- Separate responsibility from self-condemnation
- Hold accountability without annihilation
- Rebuild ethical values consciously
- Act from principle rather than fear
- Repair harm without collapsing into shame

(Litz et al., 2009; Erikson, 1968).

This ethical integration supports a life guided by values rather than reactions.

Identity Wholeness and Narrative Coherence

Trauma disrupts the life story. Integration restores narrative continuity. Survivors become able to say:

- "This happened."
- "It changed me."
- "I am not only this event."
- "My life has direction beyond survival."

(Pennebaker & Smyth, 2016; Neimeyer, 2019).

A coherent narrative does not erase suffering. It organizes it into a meaningful life context.

Growth as a Non-Linear Process

Post-traumatic growth unfolds in cycles rather than straight lines. Survivors revisit:

- Old triggers in new contexts
- Familiar fears at deeper levels
- Meaning at higher stages of complexity
- Identity as new developmental demands arise

Growth includes periods of stability and periods of reorganization. Regression does not mean failure. It signals the need for re-integration at a higher level of capacity.

The Lifelong Nature of Integration

Integration is not completed in a therapy room, a retreat, or a single season of insight. It unfolds over:

- Career transitions
- Relationship shifts
- Aging
- Illness
- Loss
- Social change
- New responsibility

The tools developed in this book of regulation, discernment, emotional maturity, agency, and contribution, remain permanent resources for navigating future stress.

Wholeness Without Illusion

Wholeness does not mean:

- Constant positivity
- Emotional invulnerability
- Absence of fear

- Permanent certainty
- Moral perfection

Wholeness means:

- Capacity rather than avoidance
- Responsibility rather than blame
- Reflection rather than reaction
- Meaning rather than nihilism
- Relationship rather than isolation

It is the ability to meet life as it is, without fragmentation.

The Integrated Self as a Stabilizing Force in the World

As survivors become more integrated, their influence stabilizes outward. Without seeking authority or recognition, they naturally provide:

- Emotional steadiness
- Ethical clarity
- Relational reliability
- Grounded leadership
- Realistic hope

Integration creates presence. Presence creates trust.

From Trauma Identity to Wholeness Identity

Early in recovery, identity often centers on what happened. In integration, identity centers on:

- Who one is becoming
- How one lives
- What one contributes
- What one values
- How one loves
- How one repairs

Trauma becomes part of the story, not the title of the book.

The Ongoing Invitation of Post-Traumatic Growth

Post-traumatic growth does not conclude with triumph. It continues as an invitation:

- To refine awareness
- To deepen maturity
- To widen compassion
- To strengthen agency
- To live ethically
- To contribute meaningfully
- To remain open to further transformation

Growth becomes not a reaction to trauma, but a way of being in the world.

From Survival to Wholeness

Survival asks: "How do I endure?"
Wholeness asks: "How do I live?"

Post-traumatic growth is the passage between those two questions. Integration is the bridge. Wholeness is not the absence of suffering, it is the presence of coherence, meaning, relationship, and responsibility in the midst of life's reality.

This is not an end. It is the way forward.

REFERENCES — CHAPTER 15

Erikson, E. H. (1968). *Identity: Youth and crisis*. W. W. Norton & Company.

Litz, B. T., Stein, N., Delaney, E., Lebowitz, L., Nash, W., Silva, C., & Maguen, S. (2009). Moral injury and moral repair in war veterans. *Clinical Psychology Review, 29*(8), 695–706. https://doi.org/10.1016/j.cpr.2009.07.003

Mikulincer, M., & Shaver, P. R. (2016). *Attachment in adulthood: Structure, dynamics, and change* (2nd ed.). Guilford Press.

Neimeyer, R. A. (2019). Meaning reconstruction in grief and trauma: Foundations and applications. American Psychological Association.

Ogden, P., Minton, K., & Pain, C. (2006). *Trauma and the body: A sensorimotor approach to psychotherapy*. W. W. Norton & Company.

Pennebaker, J. W., & Smyth, J. M. (2016). Opening up by writing it down: How expressive writing improves health and eases emotional pain (3rd ed.). Guilford Press.

Siegel, D. J. (2012). The developing mind: How relationships and the brain interact to shape who we are (2nd ed.). Guilford Press.

Tedeschi, R. G., & Calhoun, L. G. (2018). Posttraumatic growth: Theory, research, and applications. Routledge.

van der Kolk, B. A. (2014). The body keeps the score: Brain, mind, and body in the healing of trauma. Viking.

Part VII – Appendices & Resources

Appendix A – Nervous Systems

Parasympathetic & Sympathetic Nervous Systems

When respiration slows to 10 breaths per minute or slower, the parasympathetic nervous system is activated. Qigong, Tai Chi, BaguaZhang, yoga, etc. are all effective methods of exercise that activate this nervous system. These techniques have proven the test of time in being an option to remove or manage the inner critical dialogue and learn to regulate the fast paced modern existence we all experiencing.

Qigong balances breathing and promotes conditions in your body for it to be able to regenerate and heal itself. Qigong does not treat symptoms, but rather solves the problem at its root.

When the parasympathetic nervous system is activated, "happy" hormones are released, decreasing heart rate and blood pressure. This relaxes the nervous system, slows and calms all the body systems. This process then promotes regeneration through decreasing metabolic rate at all levels.

Deep breathing encourages pumping of cerebrospinal fluid (fluid around the spinal cord). This increases brain metabolism while promoting feelings of physical and mental well-being, as well as enhanced mental alertness.

A ROOT SOLUTION to COMBAT DISEASE: Activate the Parasympathetic Nervous System (PSNS)

12-18 breaths per minute average keeps us in the Sympathetic Nervous System of "Fight or Flight"

10 BPM or less activates PSNS

Fight or flight response transitions to restore and regenerate

DOSE chemicals & hormones released instead of Cortisol
D - dopamine
O - oxytocin
S - seratonin
E - endorphins

www.MindAndBodyExercises.com

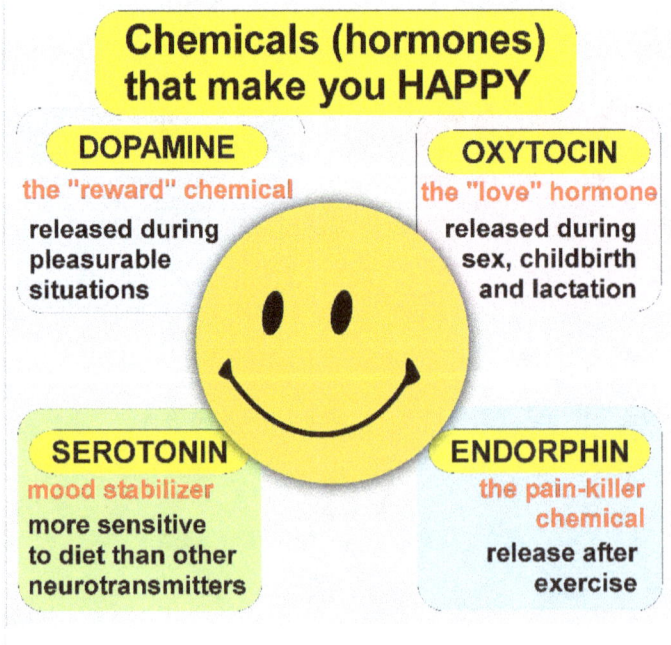

Chemicals (hormones) that make you HAPPY

- **DOPAMINE** — the "reward" chemical — released during pleasurable situations
- **OXYTOCIN** — the "love" hormone — released during sex, childbirth and lactation
- **SEROTONIN** — mood stabilizer — more sensitive to diet than other neurotransmitters
- **ENDORPHIN** — the pain-killer chemical — release after exercise

© Copyright 2018 - CAD Graphics, Inc.

NOTE: This study guide is a general reference for the exercises shown. Consult with your physician if you are uncertain of your physical ability to perform such exercises.

www.MindandBodyMartialArts.com

Too much activity within the sympathetic nervous system causes the body to constantly respond as if in the "fight" or flight" mentally eventually deteriorating many body systems.

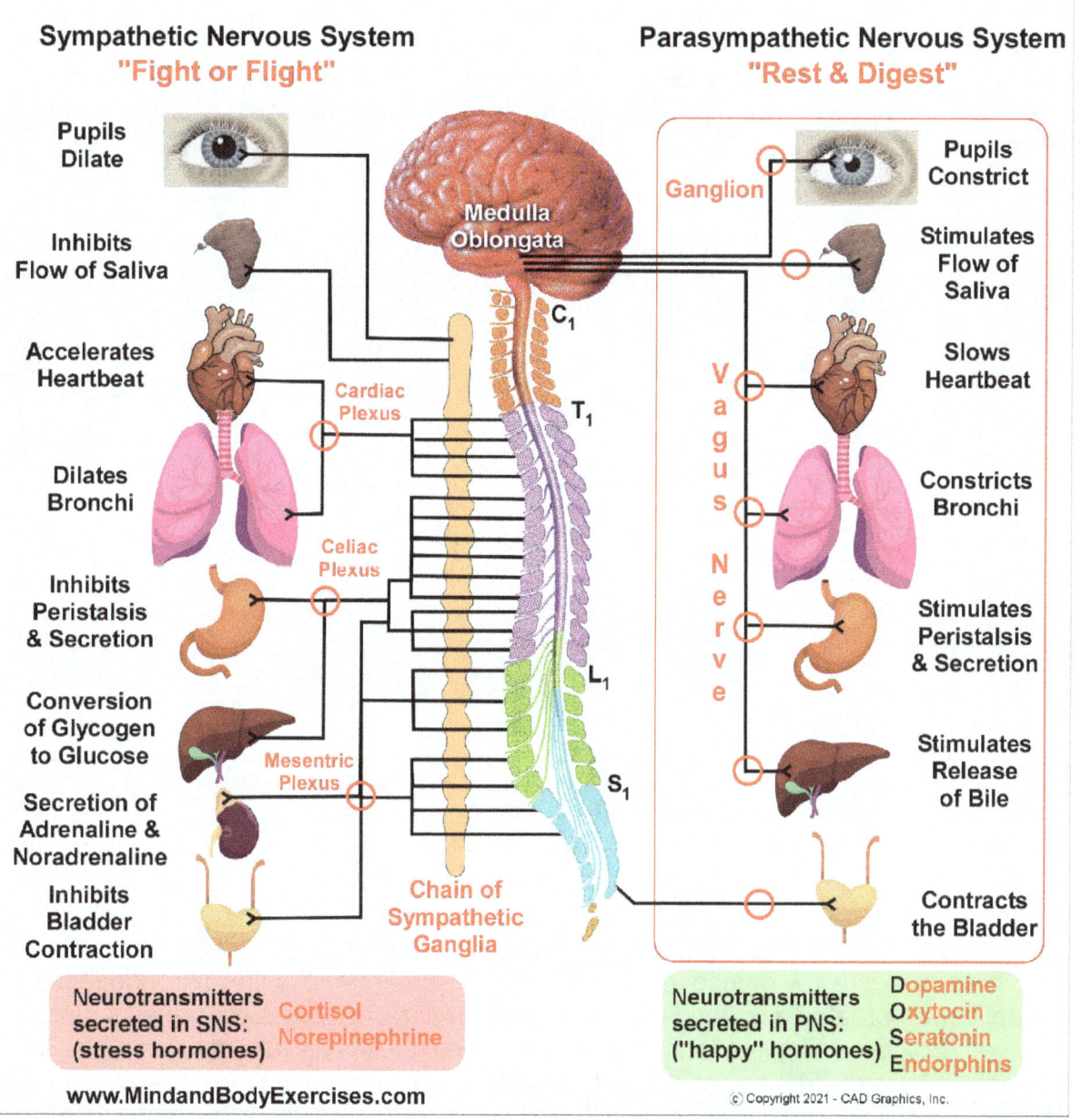

Appendix B - Box Breathing: A Method to Manage Stress

So much inner conflict, anxiety, depression, PTSD. We have tools to combat this that don't include pharmaceuticals, therapy or other harsh interventions. Americans have been conditioned (operant conditioning, B.F. Skinner) to rely upon others for their own well-being, health and happiness. Happiness comes from within. Most figure this out at some time in their life. Never for some.

Learning to manage our own breath leads to managing our emotions, which affects our blood chemistry, relative organ function and overall health. Box breathing and other methods cost nothing but time, effort and the realization that our nation's healthcare crises can be improved when people take responsibility for their own health and relative outcomes.

From a report from the White House:

"There are several indications that Americans were experiencing a mental health crisis prior to the pandemic. Between 2008 and 2019, the percentage of adolescents (ages 12 to 17) that reported having experienced at least one major depressive episode in the past year increased nearly 90 percent, from 8.3 percent in 2008 to 15.7 percent in 2019, while the percentage of young adults (ages 18 to 25) reporting at least one major depressive episode in the past year increased a similar 81 percent from 8.4 percent in 2008 to 15.2 percent in 2019 (Figure 1). Over roughly the same period, suicide death rates among individuals 10 to 24 years of age increased 47 percent. Although rates of depression were highest among adolescents and young adults, more broadly in 2019, over one in five adults age 18 or older were classified as having a mental illness, and more than 13.1 million (or 5 percent) of adults had disorders that were classified as serious because they substantially interfered with or limited one or more major life activities. Rates of mental illness were highest among those age 18 to 25, females, and those reporting their race as other..

Among children age 3-17, the most commonly diagnosed mental disorders from 2013 to 2019 were ADHD (9.8 percent), anxiety (9.4 percent), behavioral problems (8.9 percent), and depression (4.4 percent). These disorders often begin in early childhood: approximately one in six U.S. children age 2-8 had a diagnosed mental, behavioral or developmental disorder."

Deep breathing is a key component to having a long and healthy life. Through focused and deliberate breathing methods, many positive mental and physical benefits can be achieved. Box breathing is a technique to slow one's breathing rate per minute (BPM). Slower BPM allows precise self-regulation of the parasympathetic nervous system, also referred to as the or the "rest and digest" response or the sympathetic nervous system also known as "flight or fight" response. Both of these responses regulate our blood chemistry which can affect emotions as well as organ function. This technique needs to practice regularly and often in order to gain the benefits of deep and regulated breathing. One time will not do much.

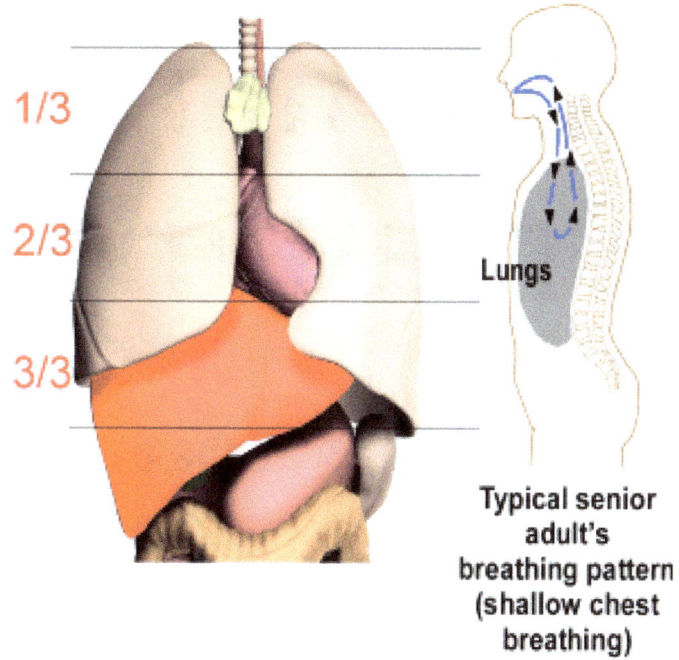

Tai chi, qigong, martial arts, meditation, yoga and some other exercise curriculum often offer box breathing techniques and many others. I have been practicing, studying and teaching these methods for almost 40 years with incredible results for myself and the hundreds of others that I have shared this knowledge with.

The "Box" Pattern

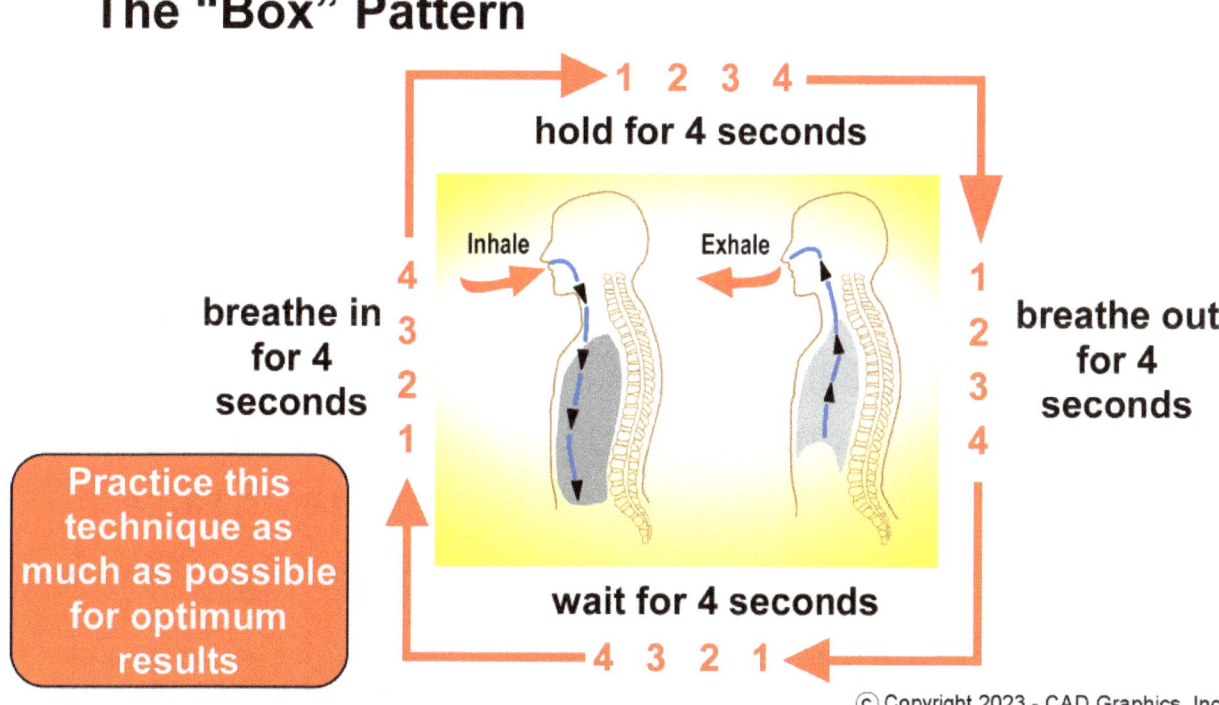

Practice this technique as much as possible for optimum results

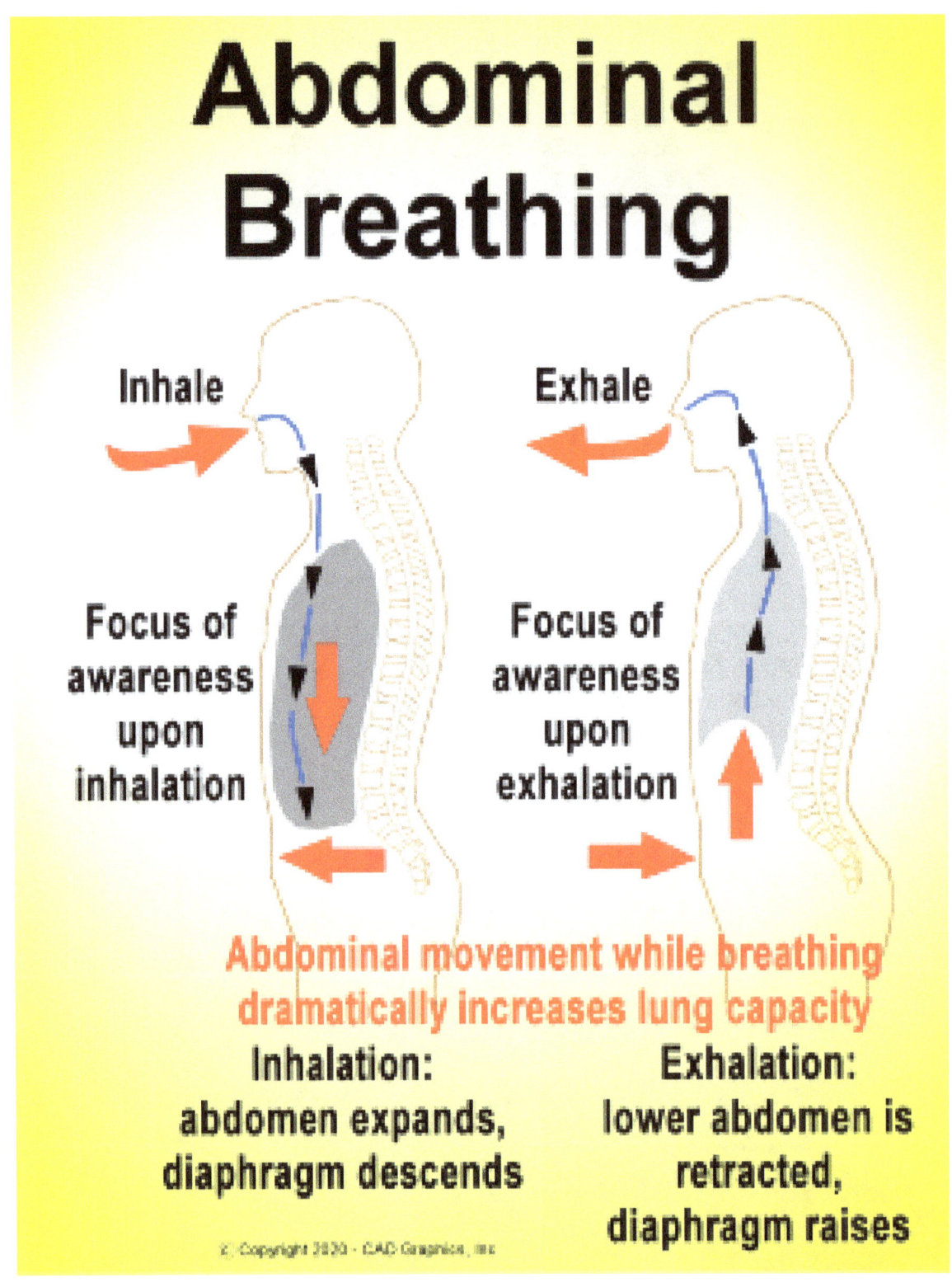

Reference:

https://www.whitehouse.gov/cea/written-materials/2022/05/31/reducing-the-economic-burden-of-unmet-mental-health-needs/

Appendix C – Other Breathing Patterns

Advanced Breathing Patterns

Correct breathing is a key to a long and healthy life. Through focused thought and breathing (meditation), many positive mental and physical benefits can be achieved.

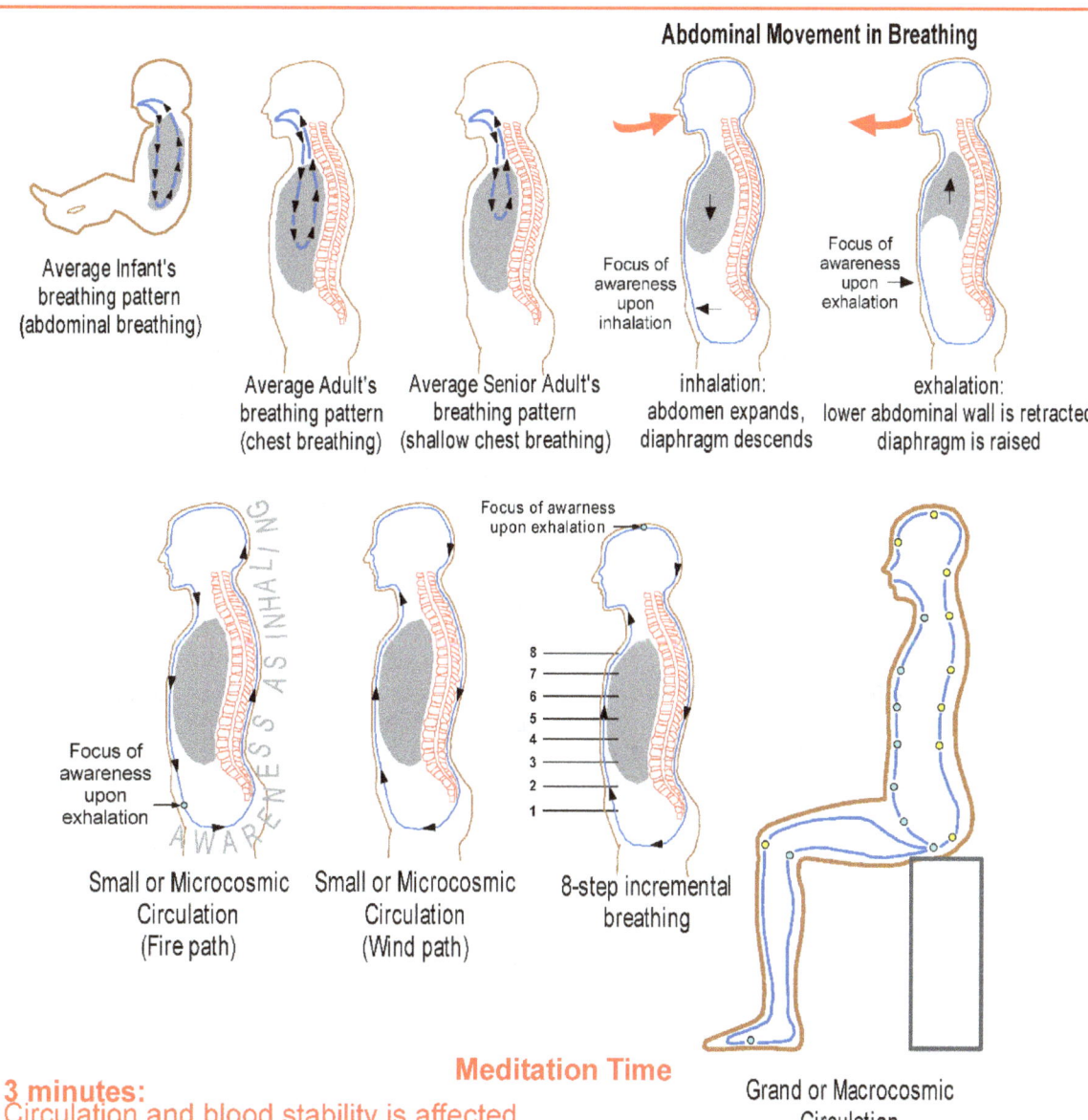

Meditation Time

3 minutes:
Circulation and blood stability is affected

11 minutes:
The pituitary and nerves begin to change

22 minutes:
The three minds (Negative, Positive and Neutral) balance and begin to work together

62 minutes:
Your subconscious (shadow mind) and your positive (outer) projection are integrated

2-1/2 hours:
Holds the change in the subconscious mind throughout the cycle of the day.

Other Benefits of Deep Breathing Practices

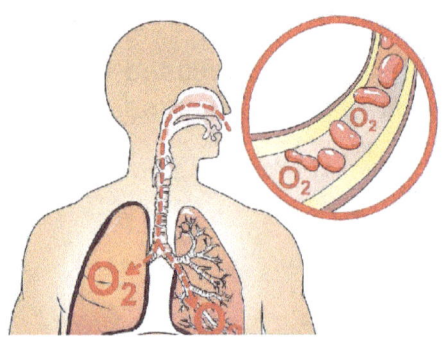

1. Breathing Releases Toxins
Exhaling air from your lungs, expels carbon dioxide that has been passed through from your bloodstream into your lungs. Carbon dioxide is a natural waste byproduct of your body's metabolism.

2. Deep Breathing Releases Tension Muscularly and Structurally
When your breathing is deep, you are getting the amount of oxygen that your body needs. When you breathe easier you move easier due to reducing muscular tension. This allows an increase in flexibility of joints.

3. Breathing Relaxes the Mind and Body, Affecting Mental Clarity
Oxygenation of the brain reduces excessive anxiety levels. Deep breathing brings clarity and insights as concentration is improved.

4. Deep Breathing Relieves Emotional Problems and Mood Swings
Regulated breathing can adjust blood chemistry which effects one's emotional state. This releases endorphins, natural painkillers that create a natural high.

5. Deep Breathing Relieves Pain
Studies show that breathing into your pain helps to ease it.

6. Breathing Massages Your Organs
Diaphragm movement during deep breathing massages the stomach, small intestine, liver and pancreas.

7. Digestive System Works More Efficiently
Breathing deep from the diaphragm massages the internal organs to function better. This regulates and calms the emotions, directly affecting the digestion system.

8. Breathing Helps Strengthen the Immune System
Oxygen travels through your bloodstream by attaching to hemoglobin in the red blood cells. This in turn enriches the body to better metabolize nutrients and vitamins. Which also helps tissues to regenerate and heal.

9. Breathing Deeply Help Improve Posture
Better breathing exercises practiced consistently, will promote better posture.

10. Breathing Improves Quality of the Blood
Deep breathing removes more carbon-dioxide and increases oxygen in the blood, increasing blood quality.

11. Breathing Deeper Improves the Nervous System
The brain, spinal cord and nerves are more nourished by receiving more oxygen.

12. Deep Breathing Strengthens the Lungs
As you breathe deeply the lungs become stronger and powerful as they are also exercised with more expansion and contracting of each breath.

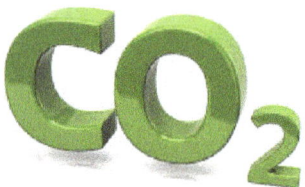

© Copyright 2018 - CAD Graphics, Inc.

13. Breathing Deeper Makes the Heart Healthier.
Breathing exercises reduce the workload on the heart. Deep breathing promotes more efficient lungs, which distributes more oxygen into contact with blood sent to the lungs by the heart.

14. Blood Circulation Improves with Deep Breaths
Deep breathing leads to a greater pressure differential within the lungs, leading to an increase in the blood circulation, thereby resting the heart slightly.

15. Better Breathing Can Assist in Weight Loss
Extra oxygen throughout the body, burns up excess fat more efficiently.

16. Deep Breathing Boosts Energy levels and Improves Stamina

17. Breathing Improves Cellular Regeneration

18. The Lymphatic System Works Better with Deeper Breathing
Increased circulation of lymphatic fluid speeds recovery after illnesses, removing waste by-products more efficiently.

19. Elimination of Waste Through Exhaling Works Better
70% of the body's waste is eliminated through the breath.

20. Self-Awareness & Spirituality Can be Enhanced from Deep Breathing
Creativity and Intuition increases when you're relaxed.

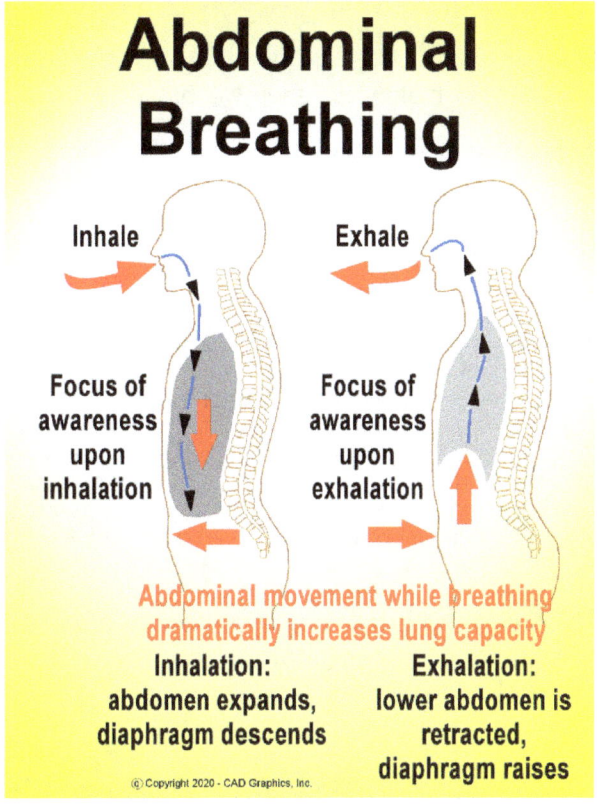

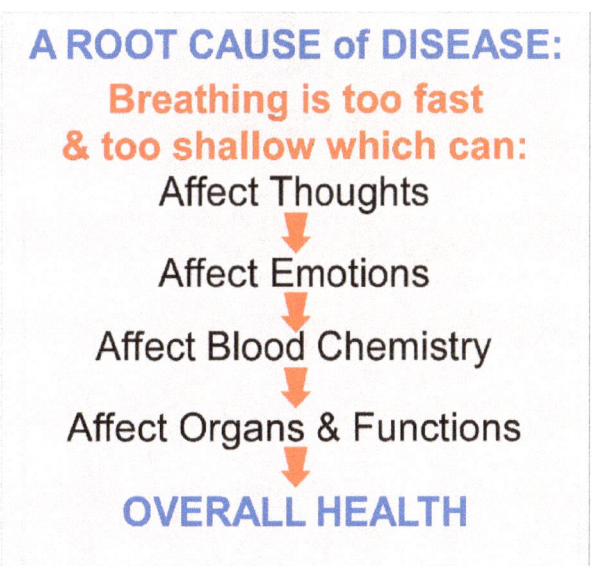

© Copyright 2018 - CAD Graphics, Inc.

Appendix D - Qigong

Qigong, Chi Kung & Gi Gong   www.MindAndBodyExercises.com

Qi, Chi or Gi means air, energy or breath in Chinese and Korean

Gong or Kung means work

Qi Gong therefore translates to energy or breath work

The human body is made up of bones, muscles, and organs amongst other components. Veins, arteries and capillaries carry blood and nutrients throughout to all of the systems and components. Additionally, 12 major energy medians carry the body's energy, "life force" also known as "qi". Ones qi is stored in the lower Dan Tien. Daily emotional imbalances accumulate tension and stress gradually affecting all of the body's systems. Each discomfort, nuisance, irritation or grudge continues to tighten and squeeze the flow of the life force. This is where "dis-case" claims its foothold.

Qigong breathing exercises can adjust the brainwaves to the Alpha state where the mind is relaxed and the body chemistry changes and promotes natural healing. Relaxing of the deep skeletal muscles, working outward. Release of tension accumulated within the muscles, organs and nerves. Whereas conventional physical exercise can deplete energy, Qi Gong helps to replenish your natural energy.

The following graphic shows how qi can be conceptualized into the Chinese ideogram of rice cooking atop a heat source and producing the wisps of vapor (energy) that we see rising above the cooking rice.

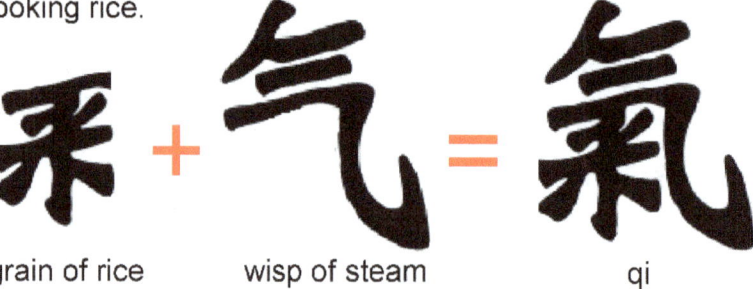

grain of rice   wisp of steam   qi

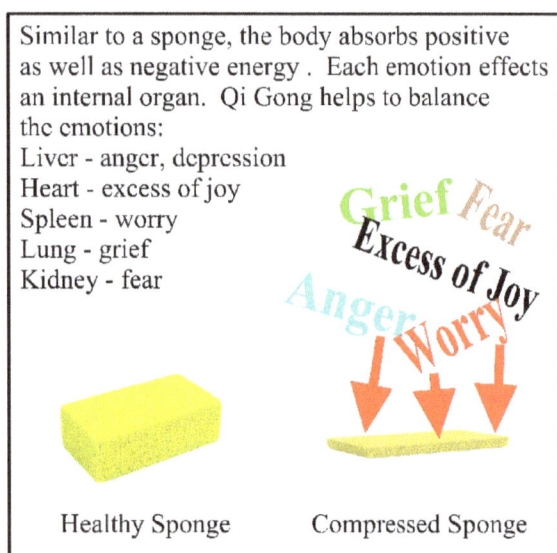

Similar to a sponge, the body absorbs positive as well as negative energy. Each emotion effects an internal organ. Qi Gong helps to balance the emotions:
Liver - anger, depression
Heart - excess of joy
Spleen - worry
Lung - grief
Kidney - fear

Healthy Sponge   Compressed Sponge

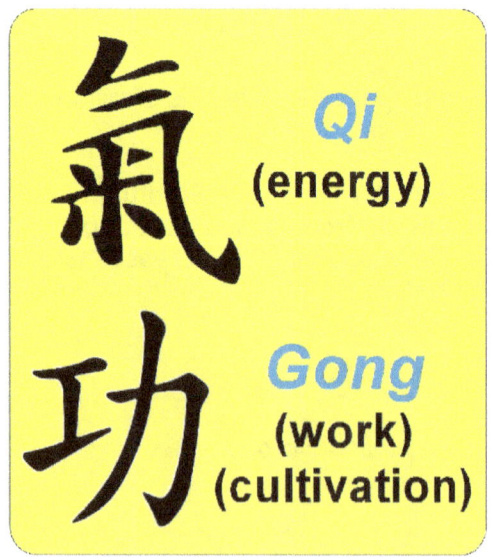

Qi (energy)

Gong (work) (cultivation)

© Copyright 2016 - CAD Graphics, Inc.

Qigong, Chi Kung & Gi Gong   www.MindAndBodyExercises.com

Neutral, horse-riding or "Wuji" stance and alignments

Head pointing skyward as though suspended by a string

Eyes closed or focus blurred

Shoulders gently pushing downwards

Lower back pushed slightly away from navel

Tailbone tilted slightly forward

Thighs gently squeeze inward

Knees slightly bent forward

Body weight 70% supported on heels, 30% on the toes

Toes lightly gripping into the ground

"Dan Tien" refers to the 3 energy centers of the body

- located at eyebrow level
- located at heart level
- located below the navel and inward

By relaxing the arches in the spine, bending the knees and tilting the tailbone forward, the spine is lengthened allowing for a release of tension and stream-lined flow of energy within the body. By aligning ones body as the figure on the left, this can be accomplished.

Lengthening of the spine

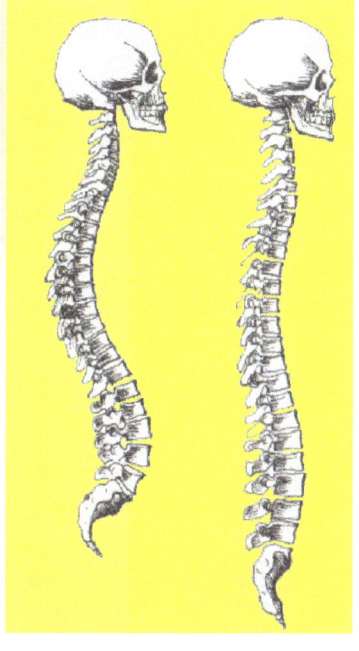

© Copyright 2016 - CAD Graphics, Inc.

Qigong, Chi Kung & Gi Gong   www.MindAndBodyExercises.com

Qi Gong exercise can change brainwaves to the Alpha state:

Alpha - relaxed concentration, creative sta
Beta - attentive, alert
Delta - unconscious
Theta - drowsy state of mind

Best Times:
- morning (calm, nature awakening)
- evenings (calm, tranquil)
- anytime (even a few minutes)

Best Locations:
- outside and peaceful
- inside and uncluttered
- anywhere possible

© Copyright 2016 - CAD Graphics, Inc.

Active Mind
Beta Brain Waves (14-30 Hz)
- State of brain most of our waking time
- Associated with stress, anxiety, fear
- Short term memory, logic
- Used for routine tasks, critical reasoning
- Stress hormone cortisol is released

go from here

Breath Management
- Focus on managing the breath
- The breath manages your emotions
- The emotions manage your thoughts
- The thoughts manage your brain waves
- The brain waves manage your hormone levels
- The hormones manage your blood chemistry
- The blood chemistry manages your heath or illness

to here

Relaxed Mind
Alpha Brain Waves (8-13.9 Hz)
- Relaxed focus
- Long term memory
- Creativity and visualization
- Light meditation, daydreaming
- Serotonin (happiness hormone) is released
- Accessed by focussing on your breathing, and quieting your mind

---

Basic Qi Gong exercise:

1) Stand, sit or lay in the position as shown to the right.

2) Try to align the body as listed in the steps on front side.

3) Inhale and exhale through the nose as the tongue gently touches the roof of the mouth behind the teeth.

4) Relax the forehead, eyebrows, eyelids, eyes, cheeks, lips and the jaw. close the mouth but don't clench your teeth. Close the eyes to take away the distractions of what your eyes see.

5) Try to picture your body in your thought as you begin a scan from the top of your head working downward towards the toes.

6) As you think of the different parts of the body, try to imagine the deep skeletal muscles releasing from the bones as if they were melting or dissolving away.

7) Continue to become more self-aware of where you are holding tension within the body. As you exhale, try to release any tension in those areas by "dissolving" it away.

8) Follow your breathe from the diagragm as you fill the lungs from bottom to top.

9) Let the stomach muscles pull inward as exhaling and bringing your thought back downward to just below the navel to the "Lower Dan Tien".

10) Continue this process as long or little as you choose, mindful that longer periods of time don't neccessarily reflect increased benefits if not performed correctly. However, most benefits are arrived at over a period of time with consistent practice.

Qigong, Chi Kung & Gi Gong   www.MindAndBodyExercises.com

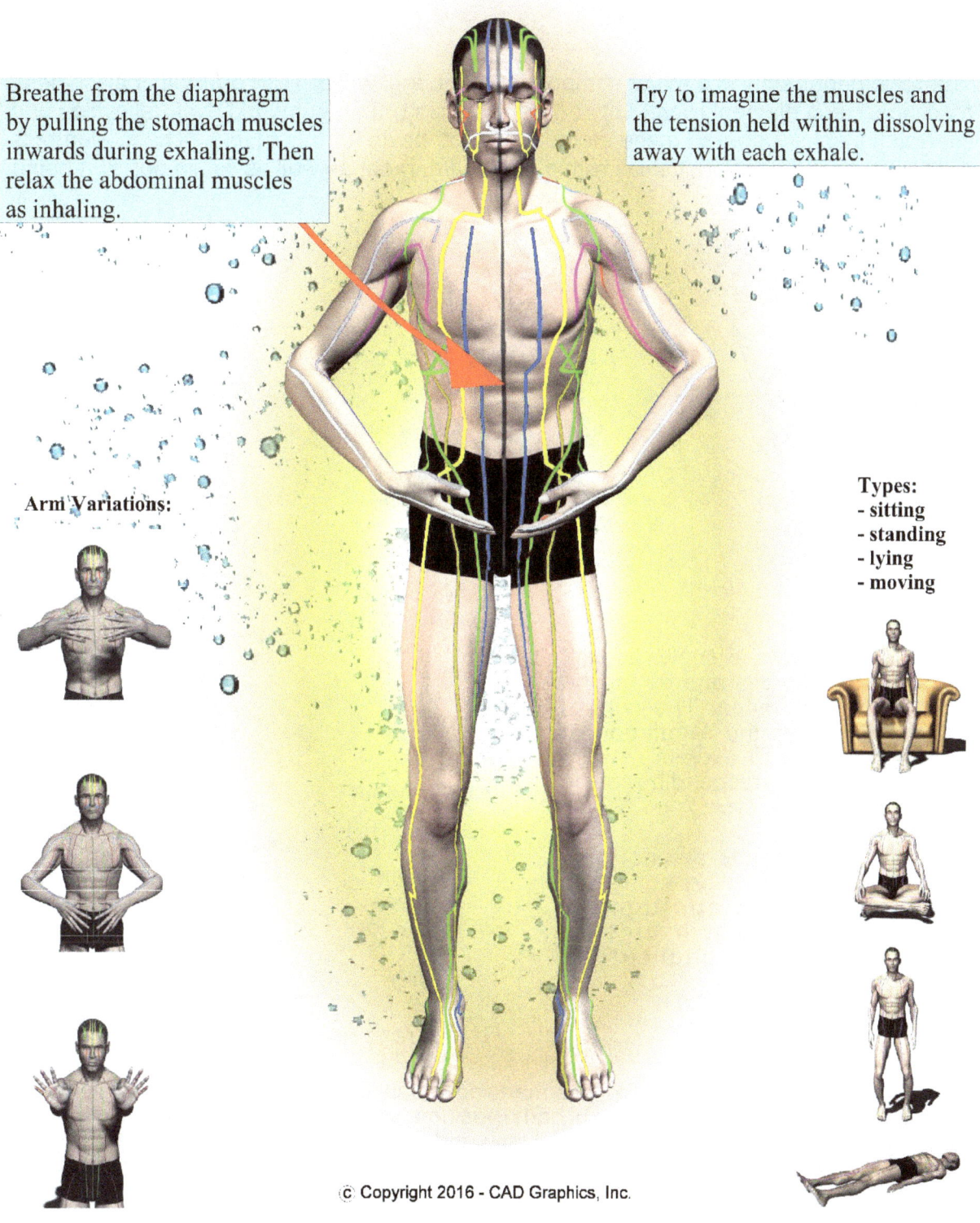

Breathe from the diaphragm by pulling the stomach muscles inwards during exhaling. Then relax the abdominal muscles as inhaling.

Try to imagine the muscles and the tension held within, dissolving away with each exhale.

Arm Variations:

Types:
- sitting
- standing
- lying
- moving

Appendix E – 5 Element Qigong

5 Element Qigong - Chi Kung

The 5 element theory is a major component of thought within TCM or traditional Chinese medicine. Each element represents natural aspects with-in our world. Natural cycles and interrelationships between these elements, is the basic for this theory. These elements have corresponding relationships within our environment as well as within our own being.

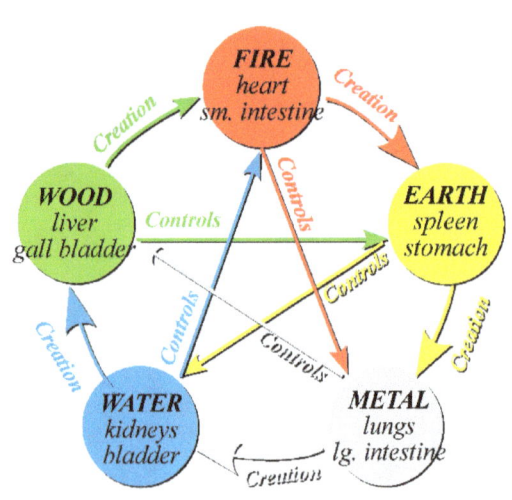

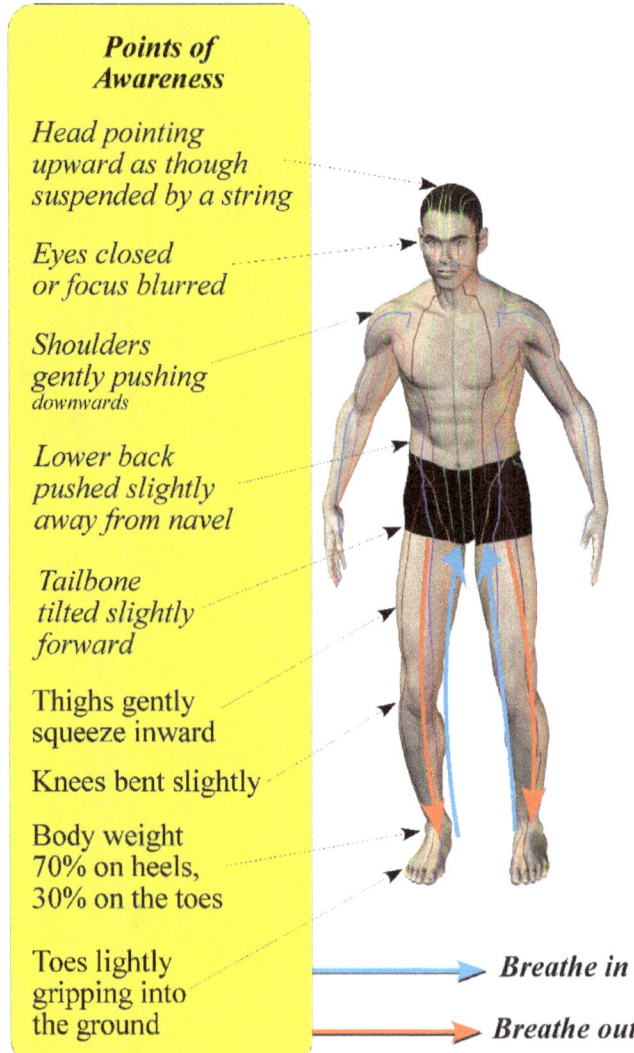

Points of Awareness

Head pointing upward as though suspended by a string

Eyes closed or focus blurred

Shoulders gently pushing downwards

Lower back pushed slightly away from navel

Tailbone tilted slightly forward

Thighs gently squeeze inward

Knees bent slightly

Body weight 70% on heels, 30% on the toes

Toes lightly gripping into the ground

→ Breathe in
→ Breathe out

In the creation cycle, as shown above, each organ provides energy for the next in the sequence. The control cycle represents the regulation of energy, relative to excess or lack thereof energy corresponding to the next element in the cycle.

Basically, the organs are not only responsible in providing energy to one another, but additionally regulating that energy in order to provide balance throughout the human body.

These exercises are designed with enhancing balance within the organs, utilizing the theory of the 5 elements. Try each body position and breathing pattern for 1 minute before advancing to the the next. Gradually add time as you are able working up to 5-10 minutes for each position. These exercises can also be practiced while sitting.

> **NOTE:** This study guide is a general reference for the exercise shown. Consult with your physician if you are uncertain of your physical ability to perform such exercises.

© Copyright 2016 - CAD Graphics, Inc.

There are twelve main medians and 8 other special meridians within the human body. Meridians are similar to electrical wires or nerves. They run from the top of the head to the tips of the toes and fingers. Each meridian is associated with an internal organ. When there is a lack of energy flow or blockage within the meridians, health problems can arise. Through proper diet, exercises and life style, it is possible to keep the chi (energy or life force) flowing through the meridians. These exercises help to increase this flow in addition to enhancing strength and balance. The illustration to the left represents the awareness of energy flow from one organ and/or meridian to the next.

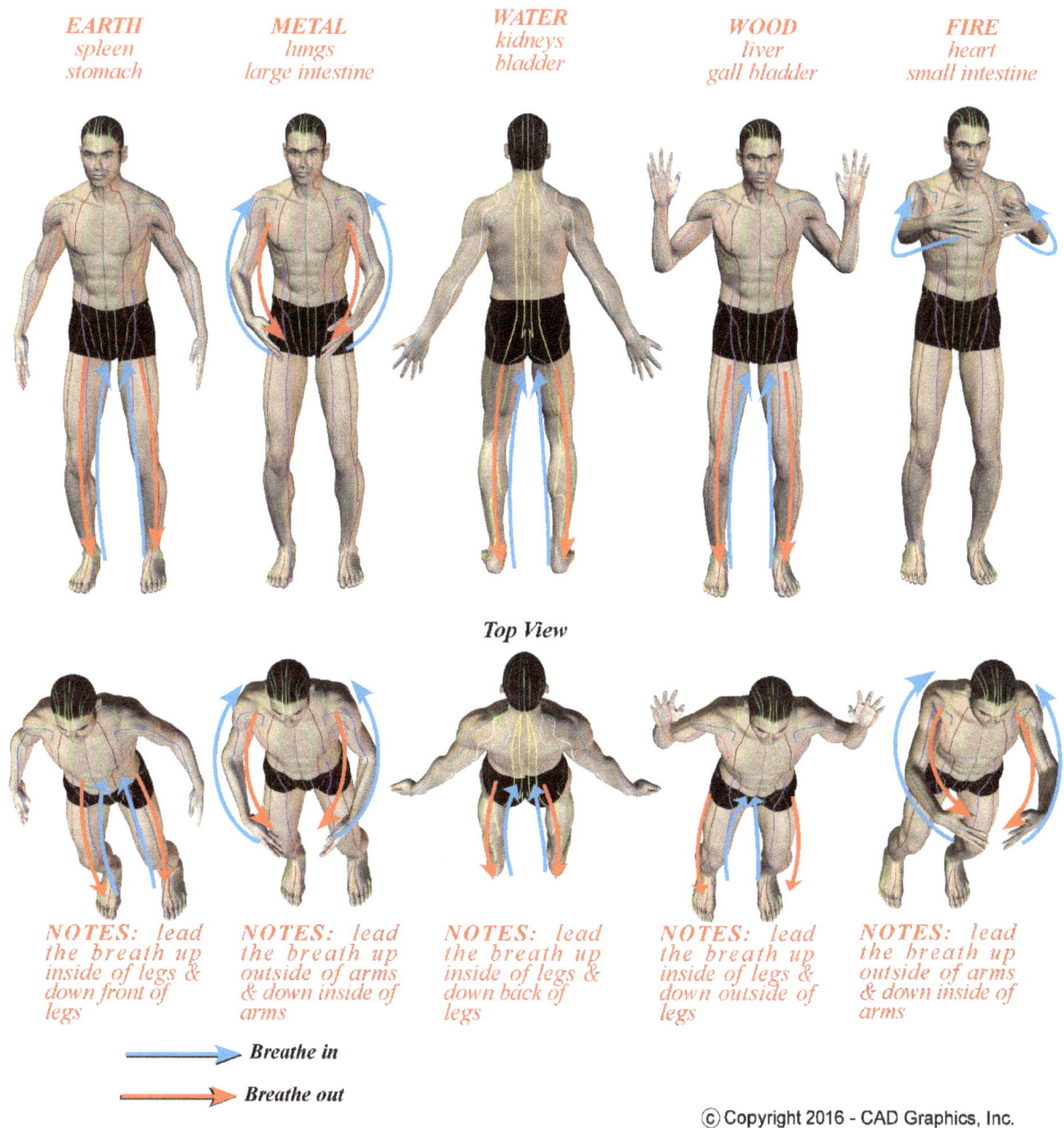

EARTH
spleen
stomach

METAL
lungs
large intestine

WATER
kidneys
bladder

WOOD
liver
gall bladder

FIRE
heart
small intestine

Top View

NOTES: lead the breath up inside of legs & down front of legs

NOTES: lead the breath up outside of arms & down inside of arms

NOTES: lead the breath up inside of legs & down back of legs

NOTES: lead the breath up inside of legs & down outside of legs

NOTES: lead the breath up outside of arms & down inside of arms

Breathe in

Breathe out

© Copyright 2016 - CAD Graphics, Inc.

Appendix F – Concept of Kan and Li

Kan & Li (water on top, fire below)

Traditional Chinese medicine and Eastern philosophy states that fire rises and water sinks within the body. Fire resides in the heart. It is inevitable that it will move upwards, fuelled by the emotional state. This causes fire to move away from the water energy, residing in the kidneys. Water sinks downwards as the essence (Jing) is not adequately preserved throughout our lives. This causes the energy of fire and water to move away from the lower energy center (DanTien) and in this way divides these two forces even more.

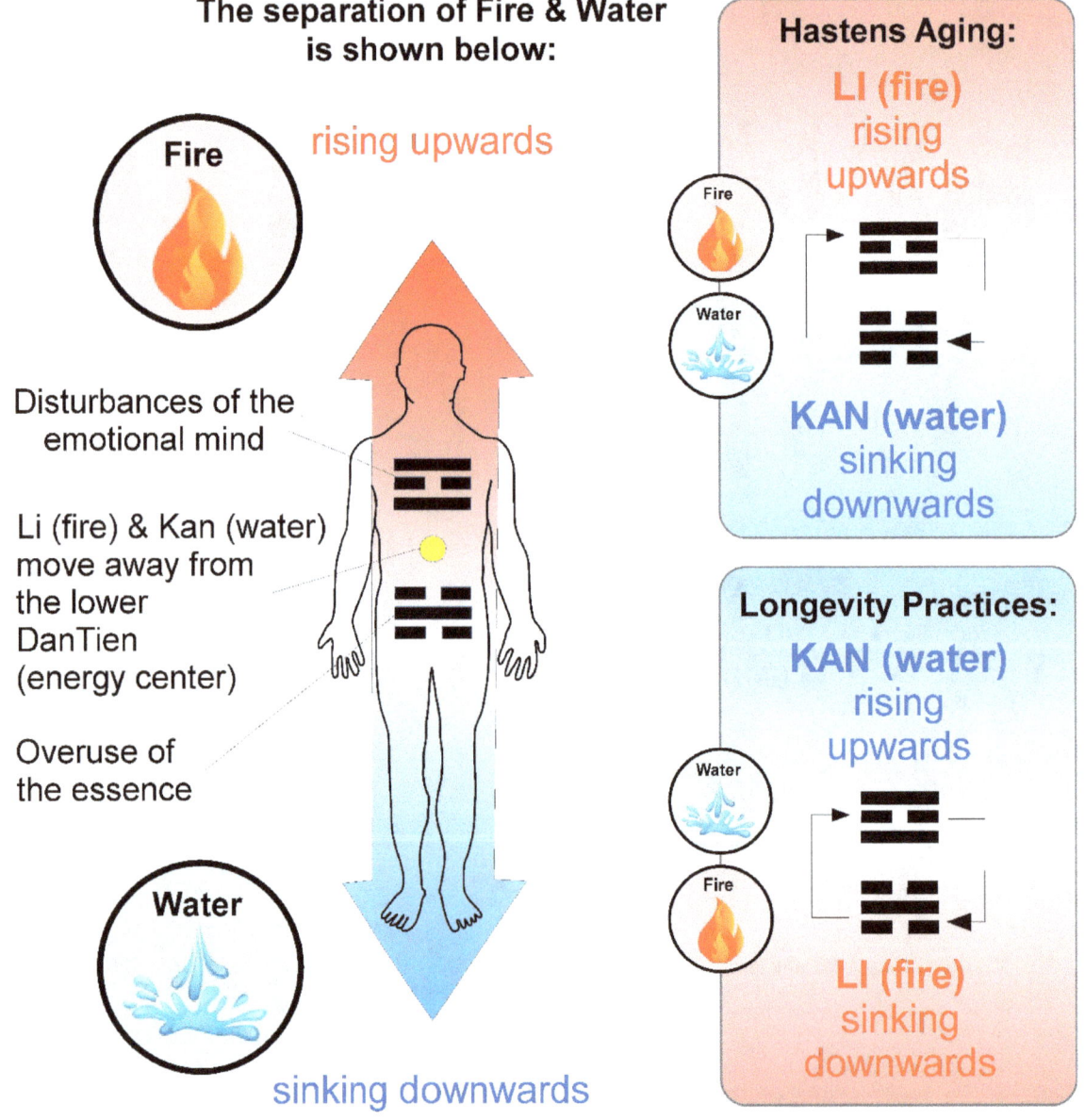

Opening the Small Circulation (Kan & Li - water over fire)

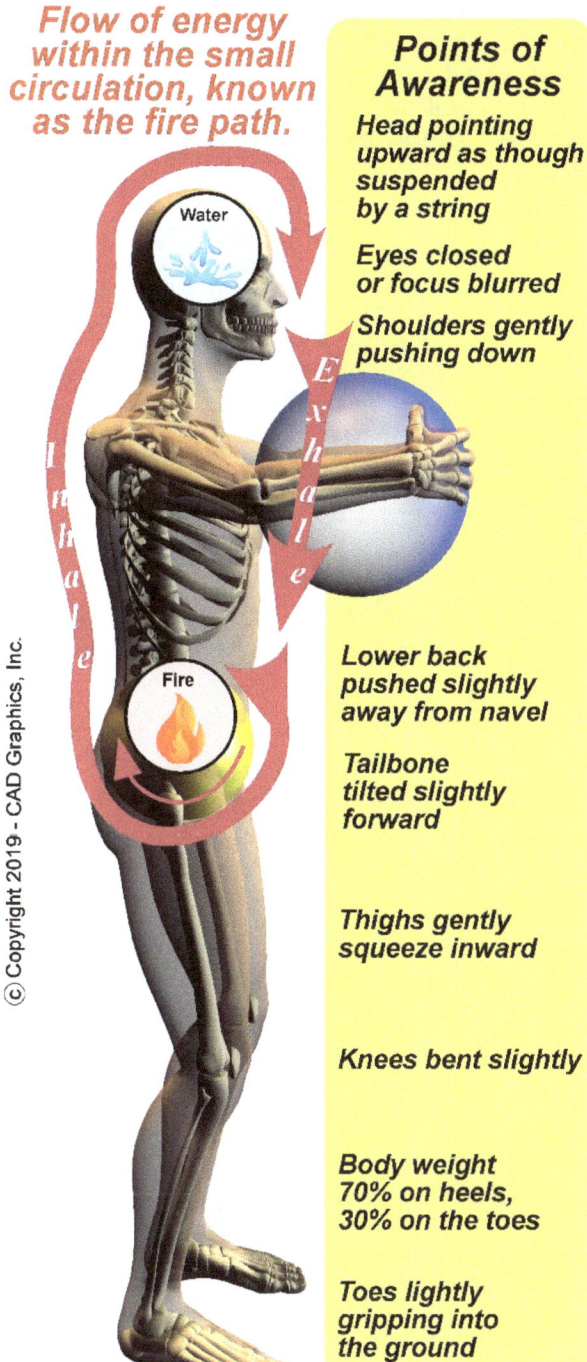

Flow of energy within the small circulation, known as the fire path.

Points of Awareness

Head pointing upward as though suspended by a string

Eyes closed or focus blurred

Shoulders gently pushing down

Lower back pushed slightly away from navel

Tailbone tilted slightly forward

Thighs gently squeeze inward

Knees bent slightly

Body weight 70% on heels, 30% on the toes

Toes lightly gripping into the ground

The Small Circulation, Small Circle, or the Microcosmic Orbit, is the practice of circulating one's internal energy (Qi or chi), within the human body. The illustration to the left represents the awareness of energy flow throughout the Governing and Conception meridians; in this case, the fire path. These meridians are located on the center line of the body and in turn govern and regulate the other meridians. This practice has been considered to be the foundation of Internal Qigong. It was a fundamental step on the path of meditation training in ancient times. Over time, this practice has gradually been lost from many meditation traditions, and its importance diminished. Though meditation is popular today for relaxation, stress relief and general health, the ultimate goal for some people, is spiritual awareness and enlightenment. Small Circulation Meditation transforms the body from weak to strong while training the mind to be calm and focused.

Visualize holding a weightless ball between your palms and chest, another within the pelvis. After conforming to the above body alignments, inhale while focusing just below the navel and following your center line between the legs and up the back, over the head and to the spot between the nose & upper lip. Exhale as following your awareness back to just below the navel.

Appendix G – Small Circulation Exercises

www.MindAndBodyExercises.com

Qigong is one way of strengthening the human body, preventing diseases and prolonging life. It includes two aspects. One being, self-training by performing postures of the human body, regulation of respiration, relaxation of the mind and body, and concentration of one's mind.

Exercise 1 — Shake the 9 Gates

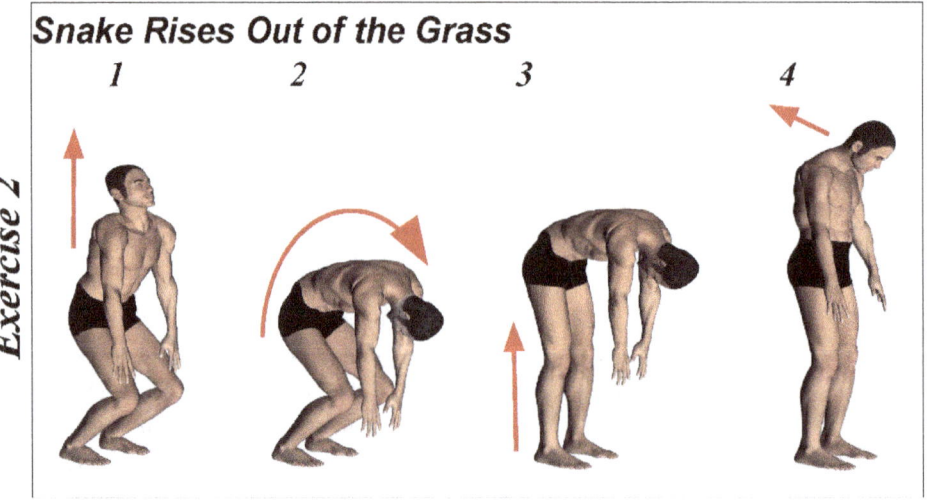

NOTES: **1-** Loosely shake hands & fingers. **2-** Continue shaking hands working your way up to elbows & shoulders. Bend & straighten knees while shaking upper body. **3-** Same motion but add gentle bouncing forward on to the balls of the feet.

Exercise 2 — Snake Rises Out of the Grass

NOTES: **1-** Inhale as bending knees as arching back, chin up. **2-** Round back as chin dips forward. **3-** exhale as straightening legs, as spine lifts one vertebrae at a time. **4-** Inhale, straighten the head and repeat from neutral position.

Opening the Small Circulation (Kan & Li - water over fire)

This aspect is to regulate and strengthen the physical functions of the practitioner's own body. The second aspect is more advanced in that the specialist of Qigong can send out their Qi externally to particular areas of another person in order to treat or prevent illness.

Exercise 3

Embracing the Sun & Moon

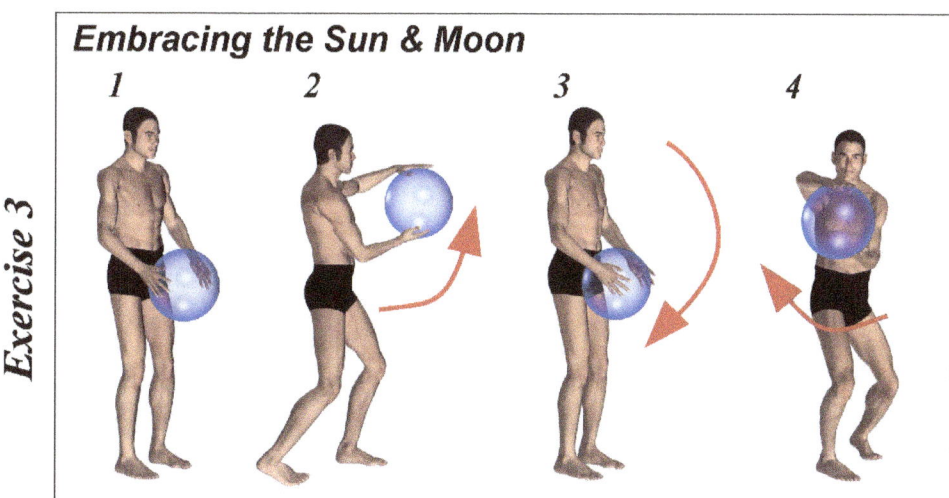

NOTES: 1- Inhale as visualizing holding a weightless ball between the palms. **2-** Exhale as shifting weight to left leg as twisting the torso to the left & lifting the arms to shoulder height. **3-** Return to center position as inhaling. **4-** Repeat as twisting to the right side.

Exercise 4

Monkey Leaps From a Tree

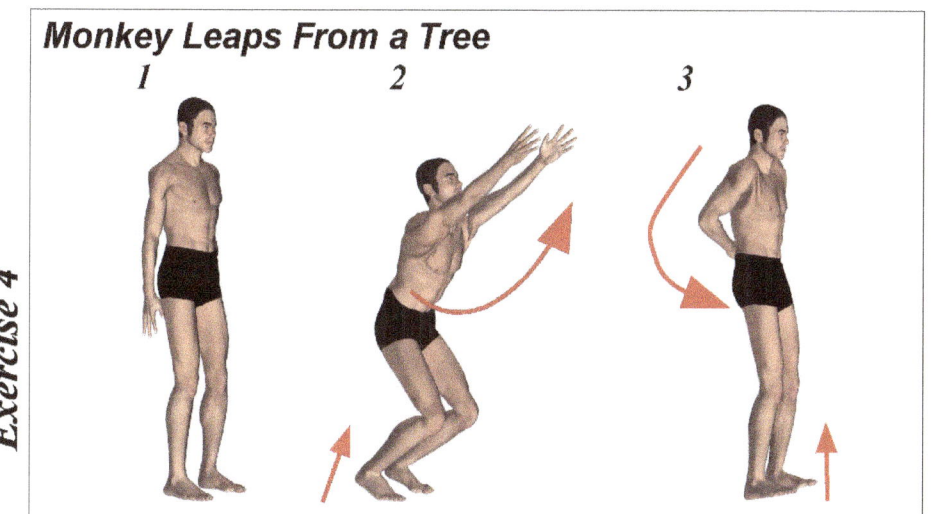

NOTES: 1- Start in a neutral position. **2-** Inhale as swinging arms forward, rock on to balls of feet. **3-** Exhale while bringing hands to lower back, round back & tuck tailbone forward, rock on to heels.

Opening the Small Circulation (Kan & Li - water over fire)

Basically, the small circulation refers to the practice of regulating and increasing the flow of one's internal energy throughout the conception and governing channels. This increase in energy throughout the body has been known for centuries to promote health and longevity.

Exercise 5

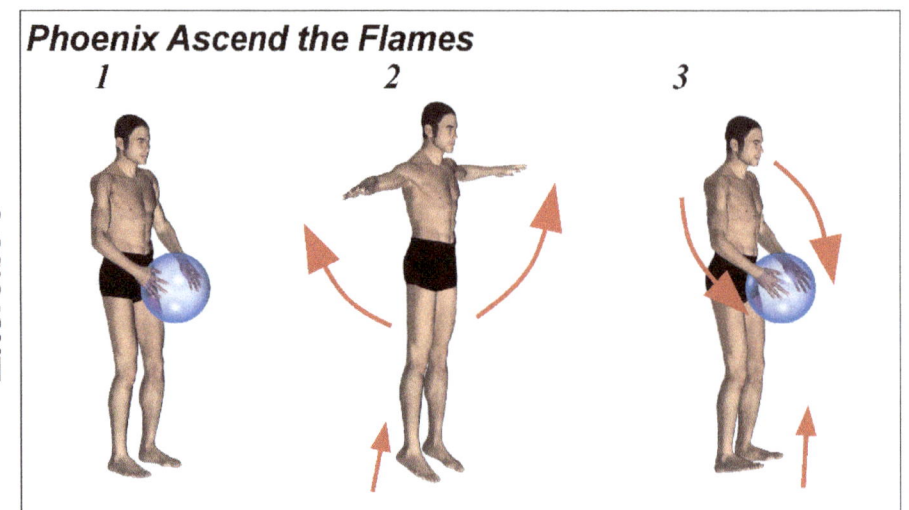

Phoenix Ascend the Flames

NOTES: 1- Visualize holding a weightless ball between the palm, rock back on the heels of the feet. **2-** Inhale as extending arms upward to the sides, as rocking on to the balls of the feet. **3-** Exhale as returning arms to start position. **4-** Repeat.

Exercise 6

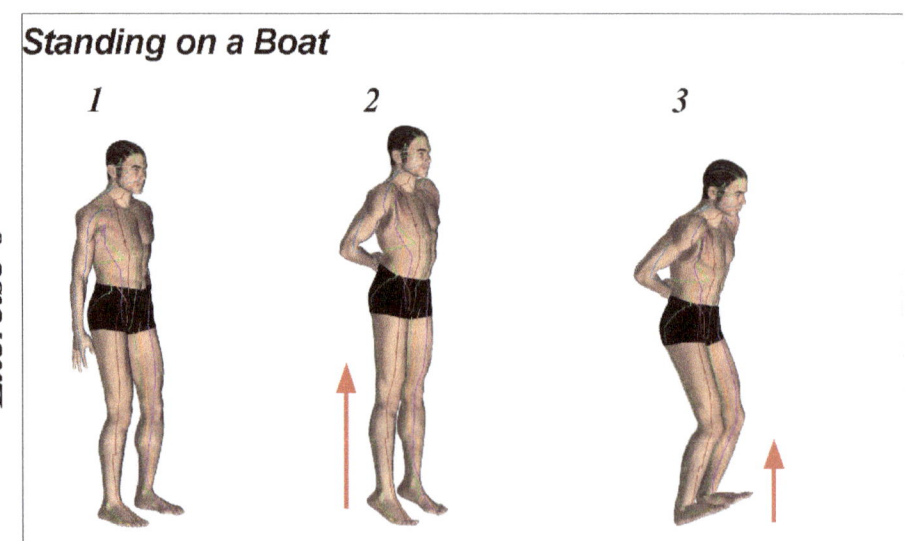

Standing on a Boat

NOTES: 1- Inhale as arching the lower back. **2-** Rock forward onto the balls of the feet. **3-** Exhale as rocking back onto the heels, while tucking the tailbone slightly forward.

NOTE: This study guide is a general reference for the exercises shown. Consult with your physician if you are uncertain of your physical ability to perform such exercises.

© Copyright 2019 - CAD Graphics, Inc.

www.MindAndBodyExercises.com

Beginning meditation training can be started by practicing breathing deeply from the diaphragm or Abdominal Breathing. The Small Circulation can be the next stage of meditation training. Eventually, one can practice the Grand Circulation Meditation, which circulates Qi everywhere in the body.

Exercise 7: Gather the Clouds to Make a Pillow

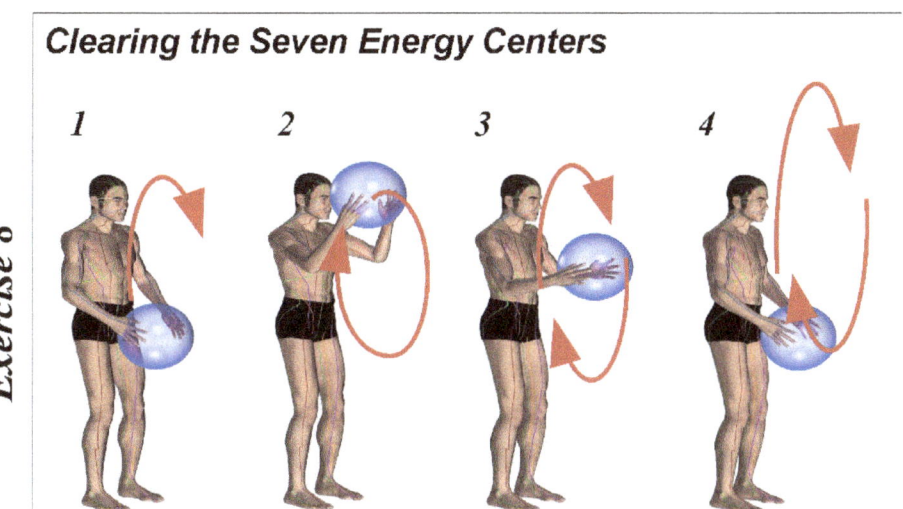

NOTES: 1- Stretch arms above the head as inhaling. **2-** Interlock fingers behind the head. **3-** Exhale as rounding spine & chin forward as bringing elbows together. **4-** Elbows & head up as inhaling. **5-** Arms push downward as exhaling.

Exercise 8: Clearing the Seven Energy Centers

NOTES: 1- Position hands as if holding a light ball in front of the navel. **2-** Inhale as guiding the arms up the front of the body. **3-** Exhale as continuing to circle the arms forward & downward. **4-** Repeat the arm motion increasing the height of the oval each rep.

Appendix H – 8 Pieces of Brocade

8 Pieces of Brocade - Opening the 9 Gates

The Eight Pieces of Brocade or 8 Sections of Silk, is said to have been composed sometime during the Southern Sung Dynasty of the 12th century by the famous Chinese general, Yueh Fei. Yueh Fei was also known to have created Hsing I, an internal style of martial arts. The purpose of these exercises was to engage the mind and body in order to balance and strengthen the body's vital functions, as well as purge stagnant energy and toxins from the body. If practiced as simple physical exercises, one can loosen their muscles, improve posture, increase blood circulation, and relax the body as well as the mind. These exercises and methods have been practiced and studied for hundreds of years to help maintain good health, prevent and sometimes cure diseases, to calm the mind, and uplift the spirit of the person performing them.

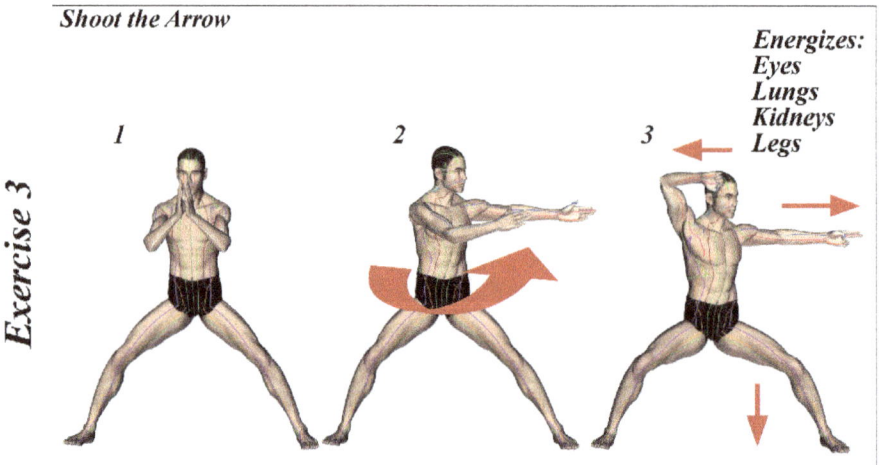

Exercise 1 — Push up the Heavens

Energizes: Heart, Lungs, Stomach, Liver

NOTES: 1- Interlace fingers and rest behind the head. **2-** Inhale as stretching arms & shoulders upward as balancing on the balls of the feet. **3-** Exhale with feet flat as leaning torso to the left side while still stretching shoulders outward. **4-** Repeat step **2**, then repeat leaning to right side.

Exercise 3 — Shoot the Arrow

Energizes: Eyes, Lungs, Kidneys, Legs

NOTES: 1- Palms press together as legs apart in a high horse-riding stance. **2-** Twist torso to the left as bringing right hand to left elbow. Inhale as drawing back right arm as if pulling back the string on a bow. **3-** Right hand in a fist, left hand has the index & middle fingers extended, while thumb, ring & little finger touch together. Exhale as sinking the hips downward.

NOTE: This study guide is a general reference for the exercises shown. Consult with your physician if you are uncertain of your physical ability to perform such exercises.

© Copyright 2016 - CAD Graphics, Inc.

www.MindAndBodyExercises.com

Ancient literature shows and explains body postures and exercise routines similar to the Eight Pieces of Brocade, but dating back roughly 2,100 years. This is important in establishing that these exercises and concepts are not a new fitness fad with little documented facts of actual benefits achieved. Some doctors throughout China, often prescribe exercises like these to prevent of heal injuries, cure illness or disease and improve overall health. This set is possibly the most popular and often practiced chi kung (energy exercises) routines practiced throughout the world, maybe my millions of people. It is just one of perhaps hundreds of different exercise sets in the vast chi kung category. To achieve optimal health benefits, these exercises should be practiced every day. Use a pace and amount of repetitions that are appropriate for your overall physical and mental condition.

NOTE: This study guide is a general reference for the exercises shown. Consult with your physician if you are uncertain of your physical ability to perform such exercises.

© Copyright 2016 - CAD Graphics, Inc.

Exercise 2

Separate Heaven & Earth

Energizes:
Stomach
Spleen
Pancreas

NOTES: *1- Place hands as if holding a beach ball. 2- Inhale as bottom hand continues to rise upward as opposite hand pushes downward from near the left hip. 3- Exhale as returning the hands to the ball holding position with the hands now opposite. 4- Repeat step 2 with arms opposite as to alternate sides.*

Exercise 4

Looking Side to Side

Energizes:
Eyes
Spleen
Immunity

NOTES: *1- Interlock fingers behind the head and inhale. 2- Reposition back of left hand onto lower back as turning head to the left & exhaling. 3- Turn head to the right as switching the arms to the opposite position.*

8 Pieces of Brocade - Opening the 9 Gates

Focusing of the mind and one's intention are key in accessing the advanced benefits available from this set. Utilizing the concept of "where thought goes, energy follows", can enhance the movement of "chi" or life force within the body. Slower and deliberate movements will greatly help improve your focus by paying attention to the body as moving exactly how and where you want to. Some traditional practitioners share the view that 100 days of consecutive practice will provide noticeable benefits well beyond the basic benefits of increased strength, flexibility and balance. Cultivating internal wellness requires some consistent effort.

NOTE: This study guide is a general reference for the exercises shown. Consult with your physician if you are uncertain of your physical ability to perform such exercises.

© Copyright 2016 - CAD Graphics, Inc.

Exercise 5

Sway the Head & Swing the Tail

Energizes:
Heart
Waist

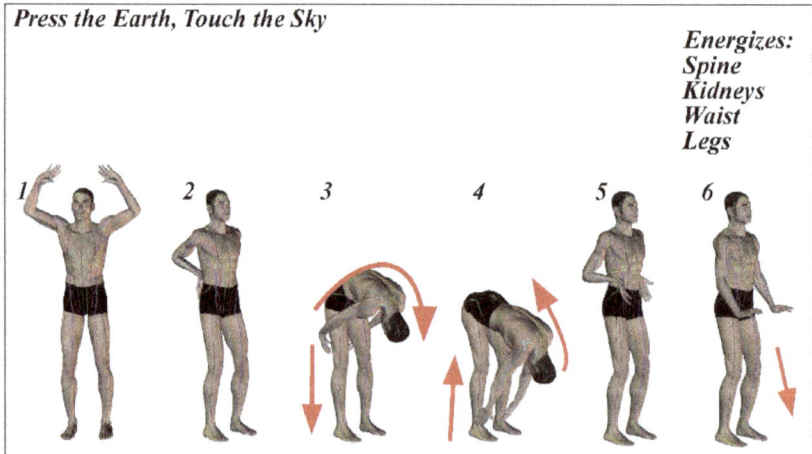

NOTES: 1- Wide horse stance with hands on thighs and torso leaning forward as inhaling. **2-** Exhale as twisting the head and torso to the left while keeping hands on thighs. **3-** Alternate twisting from left to right.

Exercise 7

Press the Earth, Touch the Sky

Energizes:
Spine
Kidneys
Waist
Legs

NOTES: 1- Arms make a heart shape motion as inhaling. **2-** Hands come to rest on the lower back. **3-** Exhale as bending spine forward as hands glide down back of legs to the heels. **4-** Inhale as straightening the spine as hands glide up the front of the legs. **5&6-** Exhale as straightening arms downward.

Anything of value worth achieving, will take some time and effort. One cannot grow a garden in one day and expect to reap the fruit without some time and nurturing. Relax as breathing deeply and naturally while doing the 8 Brocades. Sink your weight into the earth as becoming fully aware of your body and the surroundings. Relax the facial muscles and blur the vision. Perform 10 or more repetitions before advancing to the next exercise in this series.

NOTE: This study guide is a general reference for the exercises shown. Consult with your physician if you are uncertain of your physical ability to perform such exercises.

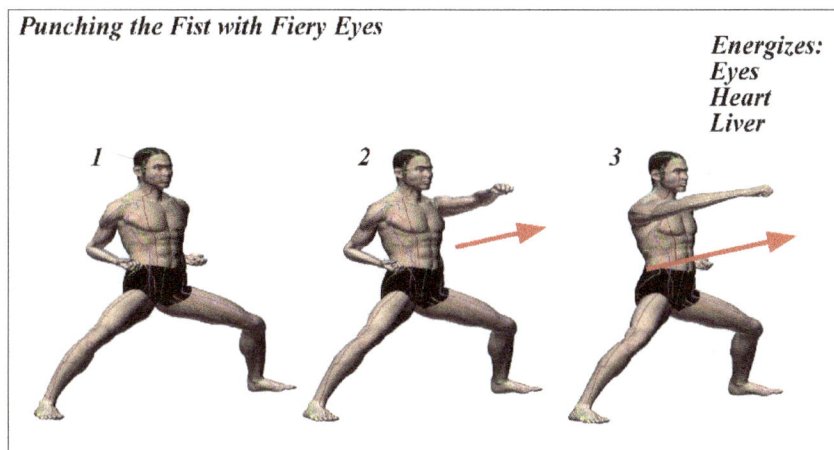

Exercise 6

Punching the Fist with Fiery Eyes

Energizes:
Eyes
Heart
Liver

NOTES: 1- Wide horse stance with arms back and fists palm up on hips. **2-** Exhale as extending left fist forward as turning fist to have palm facing down-ward. **3-** Inhale as pulling left fist back to hip as right fist repeats step **2**. Alternate from left to right arms.

Exercise 8

Lifting Up the Heels

rear view

Energizes:
Immunity
All Organs

NOTES: 1- Stand with palms on lower back. **2-** Rear view. **3-** Inhale as lifting up heels and balancing on the balls of the feet. **4-** Gently drop down to feet flat as exhaling. Repeat.

© Copyright 2019 - CAD Graphics, Inc.

Appendix I – Chamsa Meditation

Inner Vision, Pre-Birth Awareness, and the Mirror of Enlightenment

A Korean-Taoist Path of Self-Inquiry and Spiritual Return

Introduction

Within the quiet intersections of Korean martial arts, Seon Buddhism, Taoist inner alchemy, and indigenous contemplative practice, there exists a lesser-known meditative path called **Chamsa (참사)**. Translated loosely as "true reflection" or "sincere contemplation," this practice involves a series of inner visualizations that begin with the face and end with formless awareness. It guides the practitioner from physical identity, through spiritual regression, and into the vast, unconditioned presence that many traditions call enlightenment, *nirvana*, or union with the *Tao*.

Chamsa serves not only as a vehicle of personal transformation but also as a symbolic journey through layers of ego, memory, and form, toward a realization of the true self that was never born and never dies.

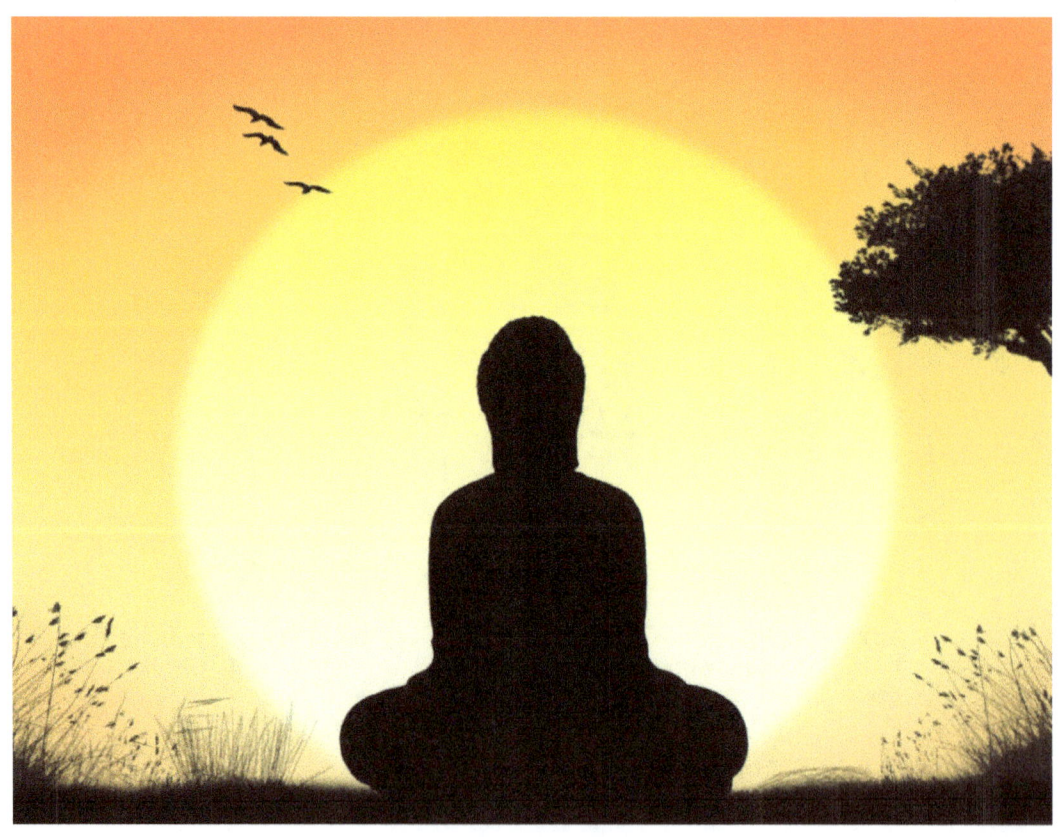

I. Origins and Conceptual Foundations

1. Linguistic Meaning

In Korean, **Cham** (참) means "true" or "authentic," while **Sa** (사) may refer to "thought," "contemplation," or "reflection" (Kim, 2018). Thus, Chamsa points to a practice of authentic inward reflection, aligned with the spiritual aim of uncovering the nature of self and reality.

2. Syncretic Influences

The practice bridges three major influences:

- **Seon (Zen) Buddhism**: Emphasizes *hwadu* (Kōan-style inquiry), non-dual awareness, and meditation as a route to awakening (Aitken, 1990; Dumoulin, 2005).

- **Taoist Neidan (inner alchemy)**: Employs visualizations, energy return, and prenatal regression to restore original spirit (Komjathy, 2013; Yang, 1997).

- **Korean shamanic mysticism**: Embraces spiritual vision, ancestral awareness, and altered states as portals to insight (Kim, 2018).

II. The Stages of Chamsa Practice

Chamsa is typically taught as a stage-based meditation, though advanced practitioners may cycle through its phases in a single session. Each stage builds upon the last, guiding the practitioner from concrete visualization to subtle realization.

Stage 1: Face Visualization

- **Description**: Eyes closed, visualize your own face in full, accurate detail, every wrinkle, mole, and asymmetry. Include features such as the slope of the nose, eyebrow placement, asymmetries, scars, skin texture, color, and even the micro-expressions of your resting face. The image should be as vivid and lifelike as if one were looking into a mirror with eyes open.

- **Purpose**: Strengthen *shen* (spirit), develop internal focus, and anchor awareness in the "mind mirror." This aligns with Taoist inner vision practices (nèishì), projecting awareness from the third eye center or upper dantian (Kohn, 1993; Yang, 1997).

Stage 2: Dissolution of the Face

- **Description**: Allow the mental image of the face to gradually blur, dissolve, or melt away without force. Observe any resistance or attachment as the image fades.

- **Purpose**: Cultivate detachment from personal identity and begin breaking down the egoic image of the self. This mirrors both Zen and Taoist instructions for letting go of attachment to form (Dumoulin, 2005).

Stage 3: Witness Inquiry

- **Description**: With the face gone, turn awareness inward and ask: *"Who is seeing this image?"* or *"What remains when the face disappears?"*

- **Purpose**: This self-inquiry parallels Seon (Zen) Buddhism's hwadu method and Taoist "reflection on the void." It shifts attention to the formless witness, revealing the distinction between perception and identification (Aitken,1990).

Stage 4: Womb Regression

- **Description**: Begin to visualize yourself in the womb. Sense the floating, fluid warmth of the pre-birth state. This visualization is not merely symbolic; it is a meditative immersion into pre-verbal, pre-identity awareness.

- **Purpose**: Return to the state of *yuan qi* and *yuan shen* (original energy and spirit), reconnecting with the undisturbed potential of consciousness prior to conditioning. This corresponds to Taoist embryonic breathing, and the process of returning to the origin (Komjathy, 2013).

Stage 5: Original Face

- **Description**: Let go of all visualizations. Abide in spacious presence. Ask: *"What was my original face before my parents were born?"*

- **Purpose**: This stage reflects the heart of Zen realization. All form, memory, and thought dissolve, revealing emptiness and unconditioned awareness (Aitken, 1990).

Stage 6: Return and Integration

- **Description**: Slowly bring awareness back to the breath, body, and senses. Open the eyes and re-engage with the outer world from this clarified state.

- **Purpose**: To integrate realization into daily life. The clarity cultivated through chamsa should inform one's behavior, relationships, and presence, aligning with both Taoist spontaneity and the Zen Ox-herding picture of reentering the world with open hands (Dumoulin, 2005; Yang, 1997).

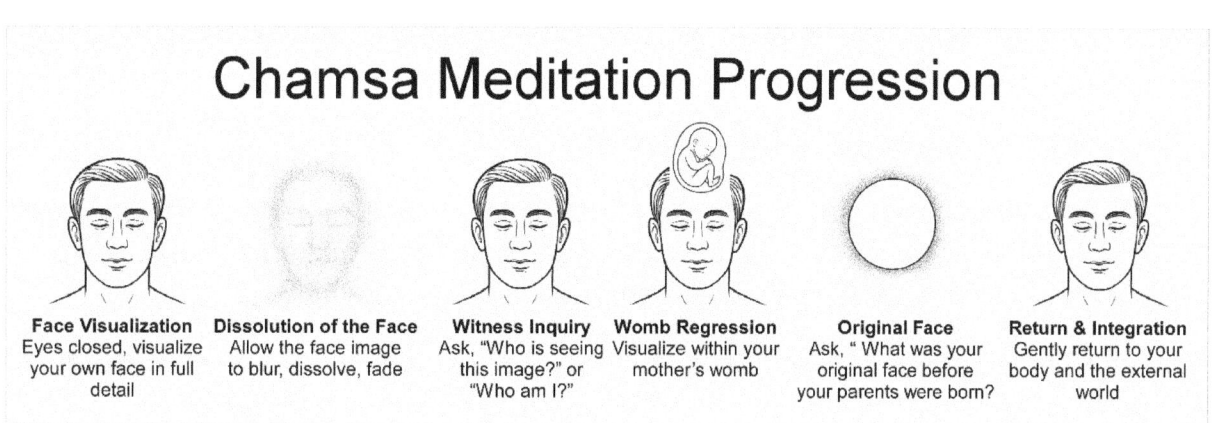

III. Practice Progression: Gradual vs. Cyclical

Progressive Practice (for most practitioners)

Stage	Timeframe	Developmental Aim
Face Visualization	1–2 weeks	Image clarity, stillness
Dissolution	1–2 weeks	Letting go, self-inquiry begins
Inquiry	2+ weeks	Direct experience of the observer
Womb Regression	Variable	Comfort with silence and non-conceptual being
Original Face	Ongoing	Insight into emptiness and non-duality

This mirrors the traditional model used in both Zen training and Taoist alchemical refinement (Komjathy, 2013; Dumoulin, 2005).

Cyclical Practice (for advanced practitioners)

Experienced meditators may move through all stages in a single sitting. This is often employed in advanced *neigong, zazen*, or during spiritual retreats (Yang, 1997).

IV. Chamsa and Enlightenment

1. As a Route to Enlightenment

Chamsa progressively dismantles the layers of self-identity. It leads to *direct realization* of formless presence, making it consistent with both Zen's gradual approach and Taoism's return to source (Aitken,1990; Komjathy, 2013).

2. As an Expression of Enlightenment

At deeper levels, the practice becomes a *reflection of the awakened state*. It is used not to attain enlightenment, but to maintain presence and live from insight (Dumoulin, 2005).

"The enlightened one returns to the marketplace with open hands." — Zen Ox-Herding Picture #10

V. Comparative Models of Enlightenment

Aspect	Chamsa	Zen Buddhism	Taoist Alchemy	Tibetan Dzogchen
Starting Point	Visualization of face	Hwadu or breath focus	Jing → Qi → Shen transmutation	Rigpa recognition
Key Turning Point	Dissolution and womb regression	"Great doubt" or koan resolution	Return to origin	Breakthrough to spontaneous presence
Final Aim	Witnessing the "original face"	Satori, then integration	Unity with Tao	Recognition of non-dual awareness
Method	Visual inquiry & regression	Self-inquiry & zazen	Breath, energy, visualization	Direct pointing-out instruction
Expression	Calm presence, embodied wisdom	Actionless action, compassion	Spontaneity, longevity, clarity	Effortless awareness, freedom

VI. Conclusion: Returning to the Formless Mirror

Chamsa meditation is both a method and a metaphor: a way of seeing the self by watching it dissolve. It begins with the familiar image of the face and guides the practitioner back to the unconditioned awareness before identity, thought, and time.

Whether used as a route to insight or a means of stabilization, Chamsa bridges Korean, Taoist, and Buddhist traditions. It reveals that the journey inward is not a retreat, but a return to that which has always been present.

"To know the self is to forget the self. To forget the self is to be enlightened by all things."
— Dōgen Zenji, *Genjōkōan*

References:

Aitken, R. (1990). *The Gateless Barrier: The Wu-Men Kuan (Mumonkan)*. North Point Press. https://archive.org/details/gatelessbarrierw0000aitk

Dumoulin, H. (2005). *Zen Buddhism: A History (Vol. 2: Japan)*. World Wisdom. Zen Buddhism : a history : Dumoulin, Heinrich : Free Download, Borrow, and Streaming : Internet Archive

Kim, C. (2018). Korean shamanism. In *Routledge eBooks*. https://doi.org/10.4324/9781315198156

Kohn, L. (1993). *The Taoist Experience: An Anthology*. SUNY Press. https://archive.org/details/thetaoistexperienceliviakohn

Komjathy, L. (2013). *The Daoist Tradition: An Introduction*. Bloomsbury Academic. https://www.bloomsbury.com/us/daoist-tradition-9781441168733/

Yang, J. (1997). *The Root of Chinese Qigong: Secrets of Health, Longevity, and Enlightenment*. YMAA.
https://archive.org/details/therootofchineseqigongbyyangjwingming1997

Appendix J – A Metaphorical Lens on Interpersonal Stress and Support

A Research-Supported Perspective on Human Energetic Influence

Human beings continuously influence one another through subtle behavioral, emotional, and physiological exchanges. Although the phrases "energy vampire" and "energy sun" are metaphors often used in popular psychology, research from social neuroscience, organizational studies, and communication science supports the underlying concepts. These metaphors capture two recognizable interpersonal patterns. Some individuals leave others feeling depleted, tense, or emotionally burdened. Others create an atmosphere of ease, motivation, and uplift. Scientific findings show that these effects are not imagined. The emotional tone of individuals spreads through groups, shapes perceptions of social environments, influences health, and even alters network-level performance.

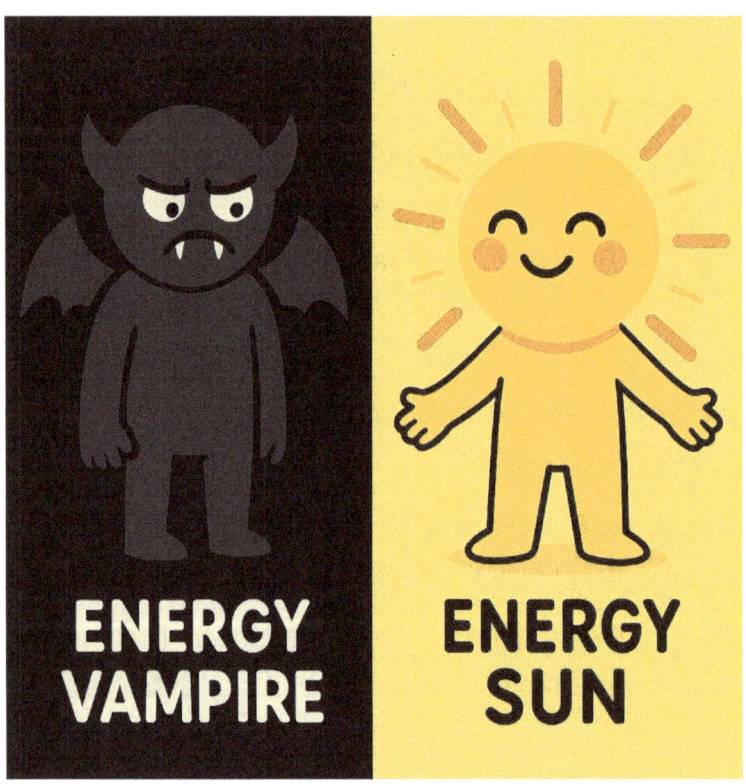

Emotional Contagion as the Foundation of Energetic Influence

One of the most robust frameworks supporting these ideas is **emotional contagion**, the automatic transmission of mood between individuals. Hatfield, Cacioppo, and Rapson (1994) demonstrated that people unconsciously mimic facial expressions, posture, vocal tone, and behavioral cues. These physical micro-responses alter the observer's own emotional state. When someone with chronic negativity enters a room, others may mirror their tension or irritability. When someone with warmth or enthusiasm enters, others tend to "catch" that energy instead.

Laboratory and field studies confirm this spreading effect. Group emotional tone shifts in measurable ways based on the mood of a single individual (Barsade, 2002). Even incidental exposure to positive or negative emotional expressions influences subsequent behavior. For instance, Kramer et al. (2014) found that altering the emotional content of social media feeds changed the emotional tone of users' own posts. This suggests that emotional contagion is so fundamental that it occurs in digital environments without direct face-to-face interaction. This highlights why trauma survivors benefit from cultivating social environments that reduce emotional overload and support nervous-system calm.

These findings support the core distinction between "energy vampires" and "energy suns." The former transmits emotional states that narrow cognitive flexibility and elevate tension. The latter transmits states that promote openness, collaboration, and psychological ease.

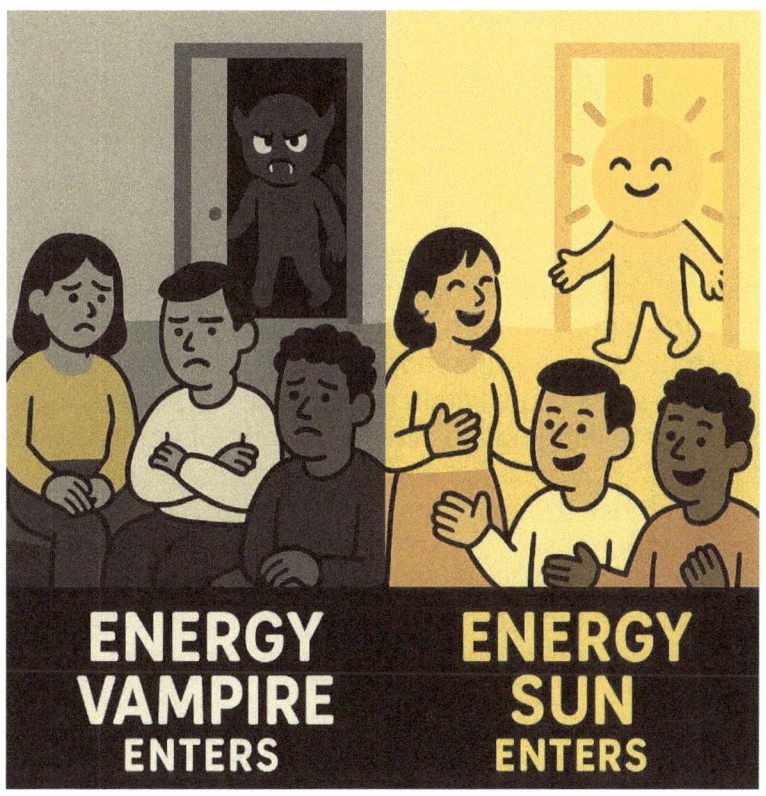

Positive and Negative Energizers in Organizational Research

Within organizational psychology, there exists a well-developed framework that parallels this conceptual language. Researchers studying **positive relational energy** have identified individuals known as **positive energizers**. These people elevate motivation, creativity, and performance among peers (Cameron, 2012). Positive energizers are consistently described as supportive, trustworthy, solution oriented, and meaning oriented. They communicate hope, strength, and possibility. Teams with a high concentration of positive energizers demonstrate better job satisfaction, higher collaboration, and stronger organizational commitment.

Negative energizers are the opposite. They are sometimes referred to as "black holes" due to their draining effect (Baker, 2003). Their communication style often includes cynicism, complaint, emotional volatility, or self-focused interaction. Research mapping organizational networks shows that individuals who are widely perceived as negative energizers reduce the quality of teamwork and the performance of those around them. Notably, relational energy has been found to be more predictive of employee performance than information flow or hierarchical position (Cameron, 2012). In other words, how someone makes others feel is more important than how much technical authority they possess.

This research provides direct empirical support for distinguishing between "energy vampires" and "energy suns" in group dynamics.

Social Relationships, Stress Physiology, and Health

The effects of draining or nourishing individuals extend beyond mood. They influence physiology. Social isolation and chronically negative relationships are strongly associated with elevated stress hormones, heightened inflammation, and increased risk of depression and mortality (Holt-Lunstad et al., 2015). Conversely, emotionally supportive relationships act as buffers against stress. For example, women who received a brief supportive gesture from their romantic partners before a stressful task showed significantly reduced cortisol responses during the task (Grewen et al., 2003). Physiological synchrony also occurs within relationships. Partners' cortisol levels often rise and fall together, demonstrating a biochemical form of emotional contagion (Liu et al., 2013). Individuals with dysregulated stress responses can unintentionally elevate the stress physiology of those around them. A calm and emotionally regulated person can have the opposite effect.

These findings again support the idea that "energy vampires" consume psychological and physiological resources, while "energy suns" replenish them.

Social Networks and Life Satisfaction

Large-scale studies show that the structure and emotional quality of one's social network predict well-being. People with more positive, frequent social contacts report greater life satisfaction, better cognitive functioning, and healthier aging (Litwin & Shiovitz-Ezra, 2011). Negative social ties predict stress, emotional exhaustion, and lower resilience.

Energy Vampire vs. Energy Sun: Comparison

Category	Energy Vampire	Energy Sun
General Impact	Drains emotional resources; leaves others feeling heavy or tense	Replenishes emotional resources; leaves others feeling uplifted and clear
Emotional Contagion	Spreads negativity, irritability, or fear	Spreads calm, optimism, and emotional ease
Communication Style	Dominates conversations; complains; criticizes; focuses on problems	Communicates supportively; encourages; listens with presence; focuses on solutions
Effect on Group Dynamics	Reduces cohesion; causes withdrawal and decreased creativity	Increases cohesion; enhances engagement and creativity
Physiological Influence	Elevates stress responses; contributes to tension and emotional fatigue	Lowers stress; promotes relaxation and psychological safety
Behavioral Patterns	Seeks attention or validation; projects blame; emotionally reactive	Shares credit; takes responsibility; maintains emotional steadiness
Social Network Outcome	Creates toxic or draining relational patterns; weakens morale	Creates nourishing networks; strengthens morale and resilience
Resulting Environment	Heavy, tense, unmotivated atmosphere	Warm, collaborative, energized atmosphere

While the terminology of "energy vampire" is metaphorical, the pattern aligns with empirically observed **toxic social exchanges**, characterized by constant criticism, excessive neediness, hostility, or emotional unpredictability. These relationships create cognitive load and drain psychological resources. The opposite pattern, nourishing and emotionally attuned relationships, aligns with "energy sun" qualities that brighten and stabilize group interactions.

The metaphors of "energy vampires" and "energy suns" are vivid representations of patterns strongly supported by scientific research. Emotional contagion explains how individuals transmit their inner states to others. Organizational studies show that positive or negative energizers dramatically influence group performance and satisfaction. Social neuroscience demonstrates that supportive or hostile interactions directly influence stress physiology. Network studies confirm that emotionally nourishing relationships consistently predict well-being and resilience.

In holistic health, psychology, and social dynamics, these insights converge into a simple but powerful truth. Individuals who enter a room have the capacity to uplift or deplete the collective environment. Recognizing these patterns allows people to cultivate protective boundaries, encourage energizing relationships, and consciously embody the qualities that make them an "energy sun" in the lives of others.

References:

Baker, W., Cross, R., & Wooten, M. (2003). Positive organizational network analysis and energizing relationships. In K. S. Cameron, J. E. Dutton, & R. E. Quinn (Eds.), *Positive Organizational Scholarship: Foundations of a New Discipline* (pp. 328–342). San Francisco, CA: Berrett-Koehler.

Barsade, S. G. (2002). The ripple effect: Emotional contagion and its influence on group behavior. *Administrative Science Quarterly, 47*(4), 644–675. https://doi.org/10.2307/3094912

Cameron, K. S. (2012). *Positive leadership: Strategies for extraordinary performance*. Berrett-Koehler.

Grewen, K. M., Anderson, B. J., Girdler, S. S., & Light, K. C. (2003). Warm partner contact is related to lower cardiovascular reactivity. *Behavioral Medicine, 29*(3), 123–130. https://doi.org/10.1080/08964280309596065

Hatfield, E., Cacioppo, J. T., & Rapson, R. L. (1994). *Emotional contagion*. Cambridge University Press.

Holt-Lunstad, J., Smith, T., Baker, M., Harris, T., & Stephenson, D. (2015). Loneliness and social isolation as risk factors for mortality. *Perspectives on Psychological Science, 10*(2), 227–237. https://doi.org/10.1177/1745691614568352

Kramer, A. D. I., Guillory, J. E., & Hancock, J. T. (2014). Experimental evidence of massive-scale emotional contagion through social networks. *Proceedings of the National Academy of Sciences, 111*(24), 8788–8790. https://doi.org/10.1073/pnas.1320040111

Litwin, H., & Shiovitz-Ezra, S. (2011). Social network type and subjective well-being in later life. *The Gerontologist, 51*(3), 379–388. https://doi.org/10.1093/geront/gnq094

Liu, S., Rovine, M. J., Klein, L. C., & Almeida, D. M. (2013). Synchrony of diurnal cortisol pattern in couples. *Journal of Family Psychology, 27*(4), 579–588. https://doi.org/10.1037/a0033735

Glossary

This glossary includes psychological, physiological, neurological, and trauma-informed terms as they are used within the context of post-traumatic growth and nervous system regulation.

A

Agency
The capacity to initiate action, make choices, and direct one's life. Restored during post-traumatic growth after helplessness.

Allostasis
The process by which the body achieves stability through physiological change in response to stress.

Allostatic Load
The cumulative physiological burden placed on the body by chronic stress.

Amygdala
A limbic brain structure involved in threat detection and fear conditioning. Often hyperresponsive after trauma.

Attachment
The biologically based system governing emotional bonding, safety, and relational regulation.

Attachment Injury
Relational trauma caused by betrayal, abandonment, or abuse by a trusted figure.

Attachment Injury
Relational trauma caused by betrayal, abandonment, or abuse by a trusted figure.

Autonomic Flexibility
The nervous system's ability to shift efficiently between states of activation and recovery. Autonomic flexibility supports emotional regulation, resilience, and adaptive functioning after trauma.

B

Boundary Formation
The developmental process of establishing psychological, emotional, and relational limits.

C

Co-Regulation
The mutual regulation of nervous systems between individuals through safety, attunement, and relational presence.

Cognitive Appraisal
The interpretation of events that determines emotional and physiological stress responses.

Cognitive Flexibility
The ability to adapt thinking, shift perspective, and tolerate ambiguity.

Conditioned Response
A learned automatic reaction formed through repeated trauma-related associations.

D

Dissociation
A protective disruption in awareness, memory, sensation, or identity under overwhelming stress.

Dopaminergic Motivation System
Neural reward pathways governing motivation, initiative, and goal-directed behavior.

E

Emotion Differentiation
The ability to distinguish subtle emotional states, linked to improved regulation and maturity.

Emotional Maturity
The developmental capacity for accountability, ethical discernment, impulse control, and relational stability.

Emotional Regulation
The ability to modulate emotional intensity without suppression or overwhelm.

Ethical Self-Regulation
The capacity to govern behavior according to internalized moral values rather than fear or compulsion.

Eustress
A form of positive, growth-oriented stress that enhances motivation, resilience, and adaptive functioning.

Executive Function
Prefrontal cortical capacities for planning, reflection, impulse control, and decision-making.

G

Generativity
A developmental stage marked by contribution to others and future generations.

H

Helplessness (Learned)
A behavioral and neurological state of passivity caused by prolonged uncontrollable stress.

Hyperarousal
A state of excessive sympathetic activation marked by anxiety and agitation.

Hypervigilance
Chronic threat monitoring even in objectively safe environments.

Hypoarousal
A state of nervous system shutdown marked by numbness and emotional withdrawal.

I

Identity Reconstruction
The reorganization of self-concept after trauma disrupts prior identity structure.

Integration
The unification of fragmented emotional, cognitive, physiological, and identity systems.

Interoception
The sensing of internal bodily states such as breath, tension, and visceral emotion.

Internal Locus of Control
The belief that one's actions influence outcomes.

M

Meaning-Making
The process of reconstructing purpose and life narrative after trauma.

Metacognition
The capacity to observe and reflect on one's own thoughts and emotions.

Moral Injury
Psychological harm caused by violation of deeply held ethical or moral beliefs.

N

Neuroplasticity
The brain's capacity to reorganize structure and function through experience and recovery.

Nervous System Regulation
The stabilization of autonomic arousal into a functional range of tolerance.

P

Parasympathetic Nervous System
The calming branch of the autonomic nervous system responsible for rest and recovery.

Post-Traumatic Growth (PTG)
Positive psychological development following trauma, including strength, meaning, and relational depth.

Prefrontal Cortex
The brain region supporting executive control, emotional regulation, and ethical reasoning.

Projection
The unconscious attribution of disowned emotional qualities onto others.

Psychological Autonomy
The ability to maintain identity, values, and boundaries within relationships.

Psychological Maturity
Integrated emotional, cognitive, moral, and relational functioning.

R

Relational Repair
The process of restoring trust after interpersonal rupture.

Resilience
The ability to recover from stress while maintaining functional adaptation.

S

Self-Awareness
Conscious recognition of thoughts, emotions, motives, and behavior.

Self-Efficacy
Confidence in one's ability to effect change through action.

Self-Regulation
The capacity to stabilize internal states across emotion, cognition, and physiology.

Shame
A deeply internalized belief of personal defectiveness often formed through trauma.

Somatic Awareness
Conscious perception of bodily sensations linked to emotional experience.

Somatic Regulation
The use of breath, posture, and movement to stabilize the nervous system.

Strategic Stress
Intentionally chosen challenge or controlled adversity used to strengthen psychological resilience and self-efficacy without causing injury.

Stress Appraisal
The nervous system's evaluation of threat versus safety.

Stress Inoculation
A process through which gradual, controlled exposure to manageable stressors increases resilience and coping capacity. Stress inoculation supports post-traumatic growth when stress is voluntary, time-limited, and paired with recovery.

Stress Response
The coordinated physiological reaction involving cortisol, adrenaline, and ANS activation.

Sympathetic Nervous System
The arousal branch of the autonomic nervous system governing fight-or-flight behavior.

T

Trauma
An overwhelming experience that exceeds the nervous system's capacity to regulate at the time.

Trauma-Informed Care
An approach recognizing the pervasive impact of trauma on behavior and identity.

Trigger
A stimulus that evokes trauma-related physiological and emotional reactivity.

V

Values-Based Action
Behavior guided by internal values rather than fear or compulsion.

W

Window of Tolerance
The optimal zone of autonomic arousal allowing effective self-regulation and cognition.

Glossary - Graphic

Abdominal breathing – effective, diaphragmatic breathing that fills your lungs fully, reaches all the way down to your abdomen, slows your breathing rate, and helps you relax.

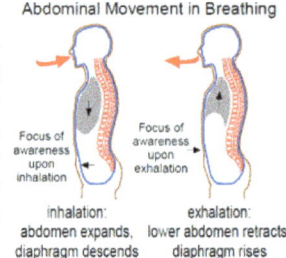

Bagua (or Pa Kua) / 8-trigrams - eight symbols used in Daoist philosophy to represent the fundamental principles of reality, seen as a range of eight interrelated concepts. Each consists of three lines, each line either "broken" or "unbroken," respectively representing yin or yang.

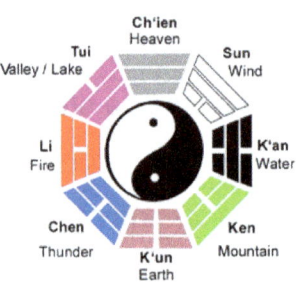

The Brass Basin – sits within the lower abdomen, touching at the navel in the front, between L2 & L3 vertebrae in the back and the perineum at the base.

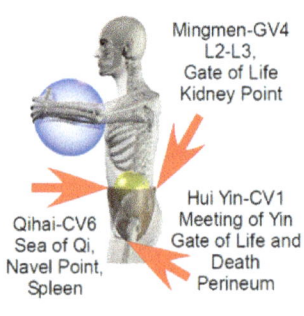

Bubbling Well - an energetic point located in the sole of the foot, slightly in front of the arch between the 2nd and 3rd toe. In the meridian system it is the same as the Kidney 1 point.

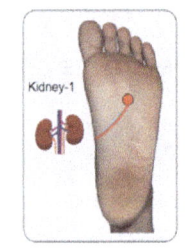

Dan Tian - 3 energy centers Lower Dan Tian (1 of 3) - also known as the "sea of qi," is positioned below and behind the naval encompassing your lower bowl and is closely related to jing (or physical essence).

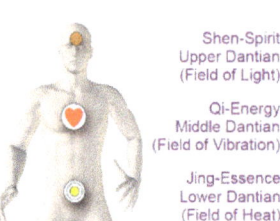

Daoyin, DaoYi, Daoist Yoga, Qigong – all names for energy exercises, with specific postures, little or no physical body movement and mindful regulated breathing patterns.

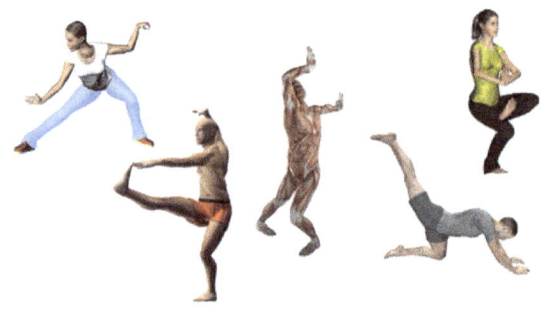

Feng Shui – translated into 'wind and water'; it is a Chinese philosophical system that teaches how to balance the energies in any given space.

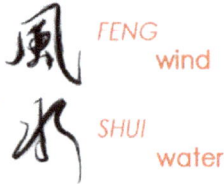

Conception Vessel (Ren Mai) – flows up the midline of the front of the body and governs all of the yin channels. The Conception Vessel is connected to the Thrusting and Yin Linking vessels.

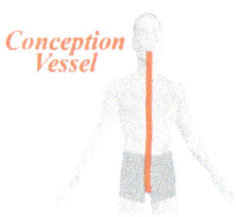

Governing Vessel (Du Mai) - flows up the midline of the back and governs all the Yang channels.

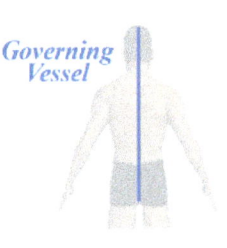

General Yu Fei – creator of the 8 Pieces of Brocade set.

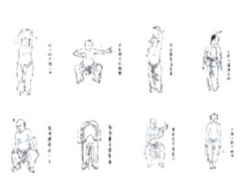

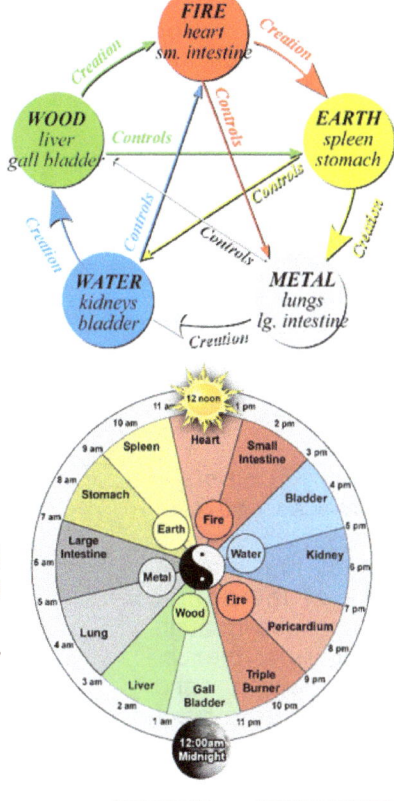

Controlling Cycle – the controlling or regulating sequence of the 5 element cycle. Wood controls Earth; Earth controls Water; Water controls Fire; Fire controls Metal; Metal controls Wood

Generating Cycle – the creative sequence of the 5 element cycle. Wood generates Fire; Fire generates Earth; Earth generates Metal; Metal generates Water; Water generates Wood.

Horary Cycle - 24 Hour Qi Flow Though the Meridians; This cycle is known as the Horary cycle or the Circadian Clock. As Qi (energy) makes its way through the meridians, each meridian in turn with its associated organ, has a two-hour period during which it is at maximum energy.

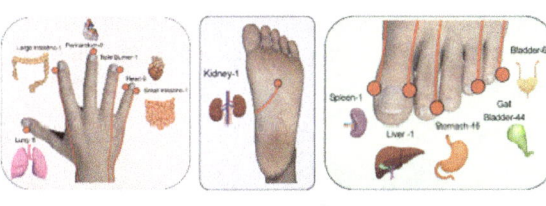

Jing Well - The Jing (Well) points are 1 of 5 of The Five Element Points (shu) of the 12 energy meridians. They are located on the fingers and toes of the four extremities. These points are thought to be where the Qi of the meridians emerges and begins moving towards the trunk of the body. These are of upmost importance in that these points can help restore balance within the energy flow throughout the human body.

Meridians - a meridian is an 'energy highway' in the human body. There are 12 meridians and each is paired with an organ. Qi energy flows through these meridians or energy highways.

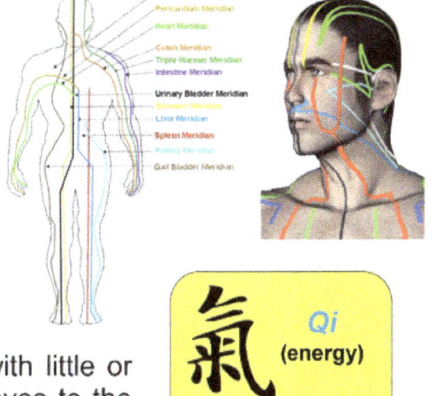

Qigong - or Chi Kung, is breathing exercises, with little or no body movement, that can adjust the brain waves to the Alpha state. When the mind is relaxed, the body chemistry changes and promotes natural healing.

San Jiao (Triple Burner/Heater) – is a meridian line that regulates respiration, digestion and elimination. It is responsible for the movement and transformation of various solids and fluids throughout the system, as well as for the production and circulation of nourishing and protective energy.

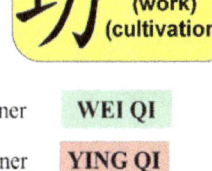

Upper Burner — WEI QI
Middle Burner — YING QI
Lower Burner — YUAN QI

Nine Gates - the energy gates in your body are major relay stations where the strength of your Qi are regulated. These gates are located at joints or, more precisely, in the actual space between the bones of a joint. The nine gates are located at the shoulder, elbow and wrists, hip, knee and ankles, and along the cervical, the thoracic, and the lumbar spine.

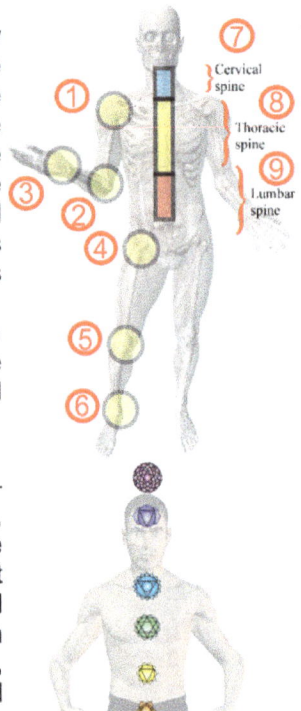

Three Treasures – Jing, Qi & Shen

Jing – (essence) the physical, yin and most dense of the Three Treasures. Think of Jing as a candle, specifically the quality and quantity of the wax.

Qi, chi or ki - (energy/breath) the energetic, vital force within all living things and it the most refined Treasure. Think of Qi as the burning flame of the candle.

Shen – (consciousness or spirit, is the most subtle of the Three Treasures and is the vitality behind Jing and Qi. Think of Shen as the light or illumination produced from the flame.

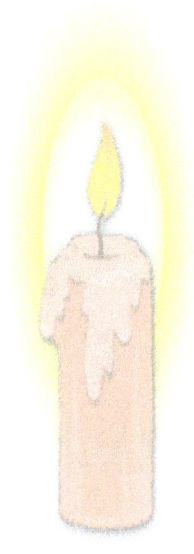

Seven Energy Centers – also known as chakras, are energy points in the subtle body that start at the base of the spinal column, continue through the sacral, solar plexus, heart, throat, eyebrow and end in the midst of the head vertex at the crown.

Six Healing Sounds – auditory sounds used for clearing internal (yin) organs and other tissues of stagnant Qi.

Metal - Hissss	Water - Chuuu	Wood - Shiiiii	Fire - Haaaa	Earth - Hoooo	6th Qi - Heeee
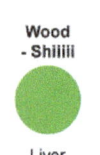	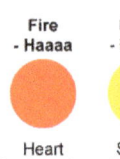		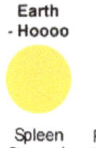	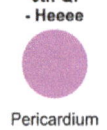	
Lungs Lg. Intestine	Kidneys Bladder	Liver Gall Bladder	Heart Sm. Intestine	Spleen Stomach	Pericardium Triple Burner

The 3 Hearts – Heart, abdomen, calves: The first heart is the heart in your chest for the oxygenation of the blood. Lower abdominal breathing is considered the second heart for circulation of fluid, Qi and digestion. The third heart is the calf muscles for re-circulation of the blood.

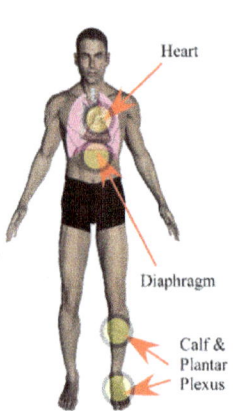

Small Circuit – the linking two energy pathways that run along the midline of the body into a cycling loop. The "fire pathway", Du Mai (Governing Vessel), extends up the back and the other, Ren Mai (Conception Vessel), down the front of the body.

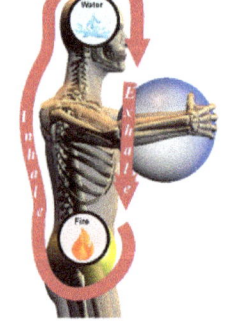

Vessels – there are 8 extraordinary vessels that function as reservoirs of Qi for the Twelve Regular Meridians.

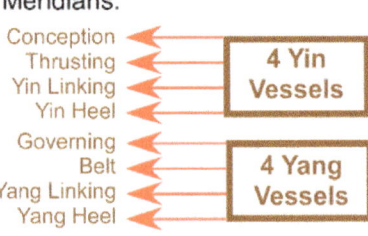

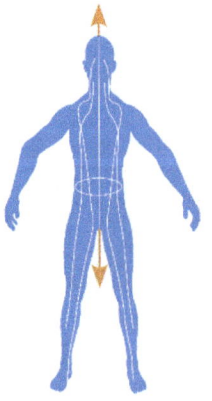

Taoism - (sometimes Daoism) is a philosophical or ethical tradition of Chinese origin, or faith of Chinese exemplification, that emphasizes living in harmony with the Tao (or Dao). The term Tao means "way", "path", or the "principle".

The Void (Supreme Mystery)

Baihui point - Governing Vessel 20 (GV 20). Sits on the crown of the head.

Wuji – ultimate stillness, the beginning of creation.

Jade Pillow – located at the top of the cervical vertebrae (C1).

Great Hammer – located on the midline at the base of the neck, between seventh cervical vertebra and first thoracic vertebra.

Yang Qi - yang refers to aspects or manifestations of Qi that are relatively positive: Also - immaterial, amorphous, expanding, hollow, light, ascending, hot, dry, warming, bright, aggressive, masculine and active.

Mingmen point – Conception Vessel 6 (CV6), the 'Sea of Qi' located on the lower abdomen.

Qihai point – Conception Vessel 6 (CV6), the 'Sea of Qi' located on the lower abdomen.

Yin Qi - yin refers to aspects or manifestations of Qi that are relatively negative: Also - material, substantial, condensing, solid, heavy, descending, cold, moist, cooling, dark, female, passive and quiescent.

Hui Yin point – Conception Vessel 1 (CV1), also known as the base chakra, is located between the genitals and the anus; the part of the body called the perineum.

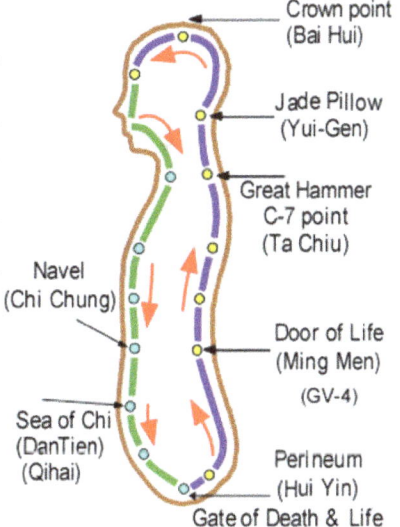

Taijitu - The term taijitu in modern Chinese is commonly used to mean the simple "divided circle" form (), but it may refer to any of several schematic diagrams that contain at least one circle with an inner pattern of symmetry representing yin and yang.

Wu Xing or 5 Elements -
The 5 Element theory is a major component of thought within Traditional Chinese Medicine (TCM). Each element represents natural aspects within our world. Natural cycles and interrelationships between these elements, is the basis for this theory. These elements have corresponding relationships within our environment as well as within our own being.

Yi – intellect, manifests as spirit-infused intelligence and understanding.

Zang-Fu organs – solid, yin organs are Zang – yang and hollow organs are Fu.

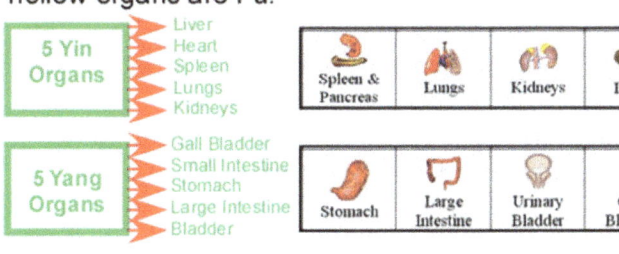

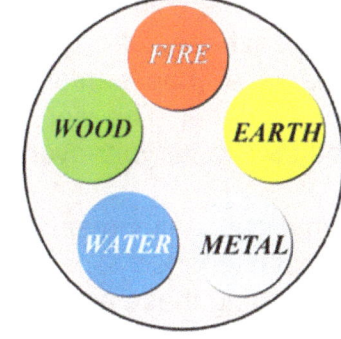

185

About the Instructor, Author & Artist - Jim Moltzan

My fitness training started at the age of 16 and has continued for almost 45 years. During that time, I attended high school, then college, and worked 2 jobs all while pursuing further training in martial arts and other fitness methods. Many years ago, I started up an additional business to help finance my next goal of owning my own school. I moved to Florida from the Midwest to make this goal a reality. Having owned two wellness and martial arts schools, I have surpassed what I once believed to be my potential. At this stage in my life, I have chosen not to open any more schools, as I found the business aspects took too much focus away from my true passion: training and teaching others.

Beyond my professional endeavors, I am also a husband and father of two grown children. I believe that we must be prepared to work hard mentally, physically and financially to earn our good health and well-being. Not only for ourselves but for our families as well. Good health always comes at a cost whether in time, effort, cost, sacrifice or some combination of the previous.

I returned to college in my later 50's, to pursue my BS in Holistic Health (wellness and alternative medicine). My degree program covered many wide-ranging topics such as anatomy and physiology, meditation, massage, nutrition, herbology, chemistry, biology, history and basis of various medical modalities such as allopathic, Traditional Chinese Medicine, Ayurveda/yoga, naturopathy, chiropractic, and complimentary alternative methods. I also studied religion, mythology of the world, stress relief/management as well as sociology, psychology (human behavior) and cultural issues associated with better health and wellness.

Most of the movements I teach and write about originate from Chinese martial arts. The Qigong (breathing work) is from Chinese Kung Fu and the Korean Dong Han medical Qigong lineage. I have also gained much knowledge of Traditional Chinese Medicine (TCM) from many TCM practitioners, martial arts masters, teachers and peers. This includes many techniques and practices of acupressure (reflexology, auricular, Jing Well, etc.), acupuncture, moxibustion as well as preparation of some herbal remedies and extracts for conditioning and injuries. I have been studying for over 20 years with Zen Wellness, learning medical Qigong as well as other Eastern methods of fitness, philosophy and self-cultivation. I have been recognized as a "Gold Coin" master instructor having trained and taught others for at least 10000 hours or roughly over 35 years. The core fitness movements are from Kung Fu and its forms in Tai Chi, Baguazhang, Dao Yin and Ship Pal Gi (Korean Kung Fu and weapons training). Each martial art has mental, physical and spiritual aspects that can complement and enhance one another. The more ways that you can move your body and engage your mind, the better it is for your overall health.

Physical health, mental well-being and the relationships within our lives; are these the most cherished aspects of our existence? Yet, how much effort do we put towards improving these areas on a daily basis?

Many have used martial arts and other mind-body methods of training as methods of learning to see one's character as others see them. I feel that I can offer the priceless qualities of truth, honor and integrity with my instruction. You must seek the right teacher for you, because in time a student can become similar to their teacher. Through the training that I have experienced and offer to others, an individual can understand and hopefully reach their full potential.

By developing self-discipline to continuously execute and perfect sets of movements, an individual can start to understand not only how they work physically but also mentally and emotionally. You can find your strengths and your weaknesses and improve them both. Through disciplined training, one not only enhances physical abilities but also cultivates mental resilience, allowing them to achieve their fullest potential in all areas of life.

I have co-authored a book, produced numerous other books and journals, graphic charts and study guides related to the mind and body connection and how it relates to martial arts, fitness, and self-improvement. A few hundred of my classes and lectures are viewable on YouTube.com.

Lineage

- Recognized as a 1000 and 10,000-hour student and teacher
- Earned gold coins through the Doh Yi Masters and Zen Wellness program
- Earned a 5th degree in Korean Kung Fu through the Dong Han lineage

Education

Bachelor of Science in Holistic Medicine - Vermont State University

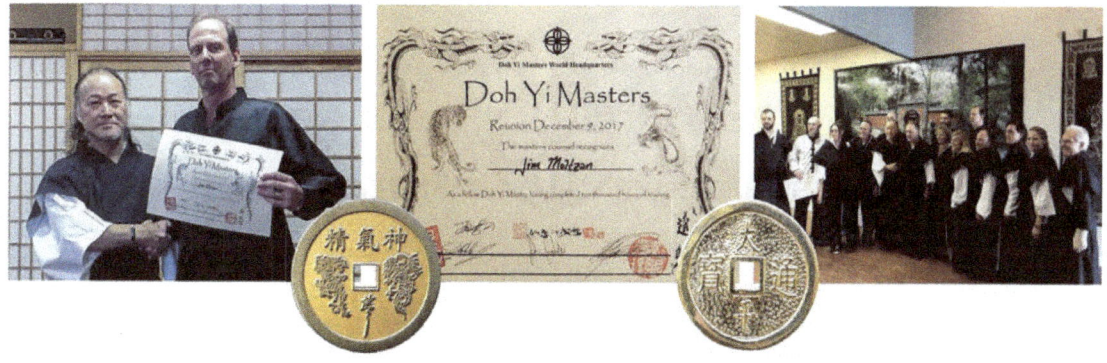

Books Available Through Amazon

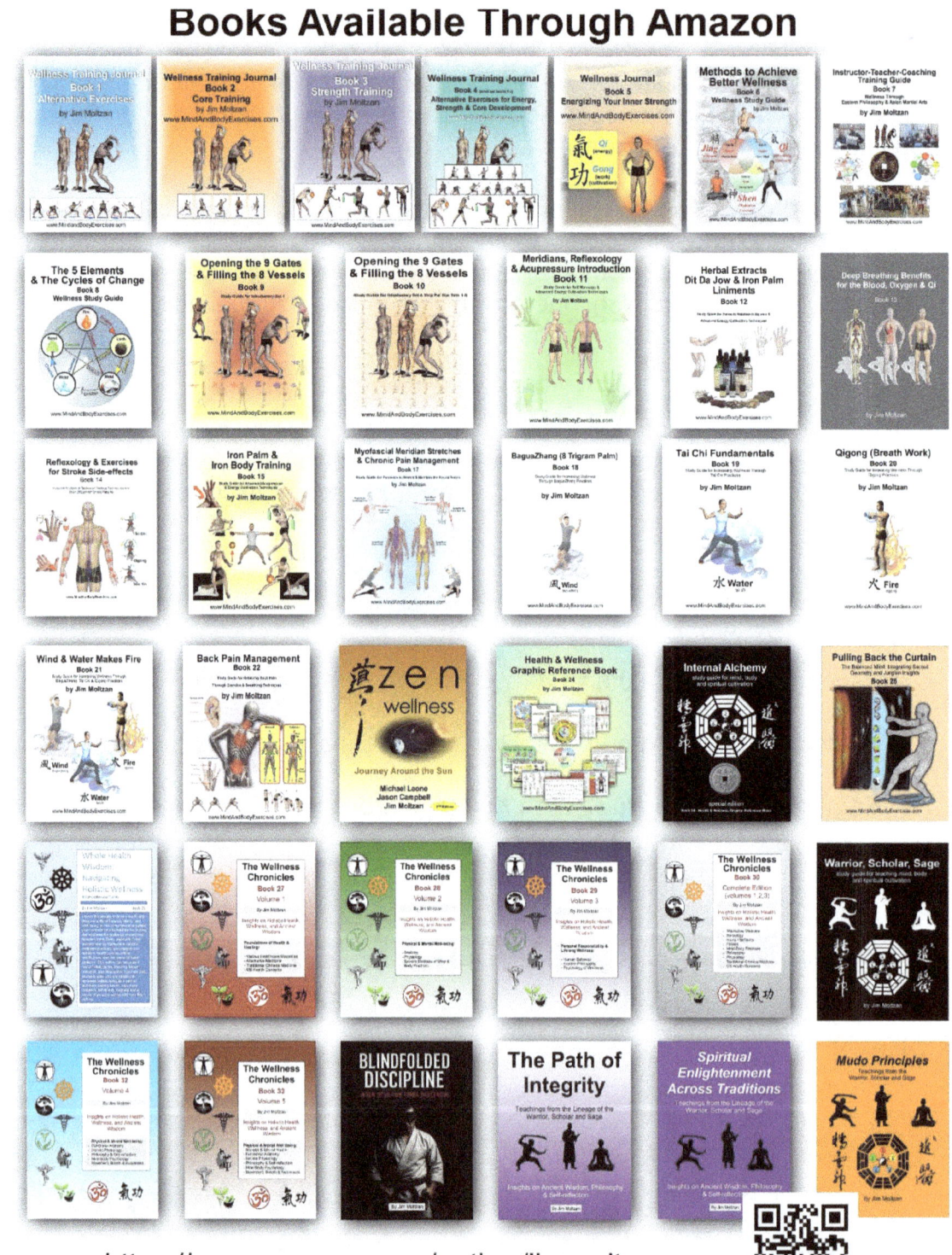

https://www.amazon.com/author/jimmoltzan

Book Titles by Jim Moltzan

Book 1 - Alternative Exercises
Book 2 - Core Training
Book 3 - Strength Training
Book 4 - Combo of 1-3
Book 5 - Energizing Your Inner Strength
Book 6 - Methods to Achieve Better Wellness
Book 7 - Coaching & Instructor Training Guide
Book 8 - The 5 Elements & the Cycles of Change
Book 9 - Opening the 9 Gates & Filling 8 Vessels-Intro Set 1
Book 10 - Opening the 9 Gates & Filling 8 Vessels-sets 1 to 8
Book 11 - Meridians, Reflexology & Acupressure
Book 12 - Herbal Extracts, Dit Da Jow & Iron Palm Liniments
Book 13 - Deep Breathing Benefits for the Blood, Oxygen & Qi
Book 14 - Reflexology for Stroke Side Effects:
Book 15 - Iron Body & Iron Palm
Book 17 - Fascial Train Stretches & Chronic Pain Management
Book 18 - BaguaZhang
Book 19 - Tai Chi Fundamentals
Book 20 - Qigong (breath-work)
Book 21 - Wind & Water Make Fire
Book 22 - Back Pain Management
Book 23 - Journey Around the Sun-2nd Edition
Book 24 - Graphic Reference Book
Book 25 - Pulling Back the Curtain
Book 26 - Whole Health Wisdom: Navigating Holistic Wellness
Book 27 - The Wellness Chronicles (volume 1)
Book 28 - The Wellness Chronicles (volume 2)
Book 29 - The Wellness Chronicles (volume 3)
Book 30 - The Wellness Chronicles (complete edition, volumes 1-3)
Book 31 - Warrior, Scholar, Sage
Book 32 - The Wellness Chronicles (volume 4)
Book 33 - The Wellness Chronicles (volume 5)
Book 34 - Blindfolded Discipline
Book 35 - The Path of Integrity
Book 36 - Spiritual Enlightenment Across Traditions

Contacts

For more information regarding charts, products, classes and instruction:

www.MindAndBodyExercises.com
info@MindAndBodyExercises.com

www.youtube.com/c/MindandBodyExercises
www.MindAndBodyExercises.wordpress.com

407-234-0119

Social Media:

Facebook:	MindAndBodyExercises
Instagram:	MindAndBodyExercises
Twitter:	MindAndBodyExercise

Jim Moltzan - Mind and Body Exercises
522 Hunt Club Blvd. #305
Apopka, FL 32703

Website

Blog

YouTube Channel